Honey Bee Veterinary Medicine

Editors

JEFFREY R. APPLEGATE Jr
BRITTENY KYLE

VETERINARY CLINICS
OF NORTH AMERICA:
FOOD ANIMAL PRACTICE

www.vetfood.theclinics.com

Consulting Editor
ROBERT A. SMITH

November 2021 • Volume 37 • Number 3

ELSEVIER

1600 John F. Kennedy Boulevard • Suite 1800 • Philadelphia, Pennsylvania, 19103-2899

http://www.vetfood.theclinics.com

VETERINARY CLINICS OF NORTH AMERICA: FOOD ANIMAL PRACTICE Volume 37, Number 3
November 2021 ISSN 0749-0720, ISBN-13: 978-0-323-89686-3

Editor: Katerina Heidhausen
Developmental Editor: Axell Ivan Jade M. Purificacion

Veterinary Clinics of North America: Food Animal Practice (ISSN 0749-0720) is published in March, July, and November by Elsevier Inc., 360 Park Avenue South, New York, NY 10010-1710. Subscription prices are $262.00 per year (domestic individuals), $628.00 per year (domestic institutions), $100.00 per year (domestic students/residents), $283.00 per year (Canadian individuals), $672.00 per year (Canadian institutions), $335.00 per year (international individuals), $672.00 per year (international institutions), $100.00 per year (Canadian students), and $165.00 (international students). To receive student/resident rate, orders must be accompanied by name of affiliated institution, date of term, and the signature of program/residency coordinator on institution letterhead. *Clinics* subscription prices. All prices are subject to change without notice. **POSTMASTER:** Send address changes to *Veterinary Clinics of North America: Food Animal Practice*, Elsevier Health Sciences Division, Subscription Customer Service, 3251 Riverport Lane, Maryland Heights, MO 63043. Customer Service (orders, claims, online, change of address): Elsevier Health Sciences Division, Subscription **Customer Service, 3251 Riverport Lane, Maryland Heights, MO 63043. Tel: 1-800-654-2452 (U.S. and Canada); 314-447-8871 (ouside U.S. and Canada). Fax: 314-447-8029. E-mail: journalscustomerservice-usa@elsevier.com (for print support); journalsonlinesupport-usa@elsevier.com (for online support).**

Reprints. For copies of 100 or more, of articles in this publication, please contact the Commercial Reprints Department, Elsevier Inc., 360 Park Avenue South, New York, NY 10010-1710. Tel.: 212-633-3874; Fax: 212-633-3820; E-mail: reprints@elsevier.com.

Veterinary Clinics of North America: Food Animal Practice is covered in *Current Contents/Agriculture, Biology and Environmental Sciences, MEDLINE/PubMed (Index Medicus), and Excerpta Medica.*

Contributors

CONSULTING EDITOR

ROBERT A. SMITH, DVM, MS
Diplomate, American Board of Veterinary Practitioners; Veterinary Research and Consulting Services, LLC, Greeley, Colorado, USA; Veterinary Research and Consulting Services, LLC, Stillwater, Oklahoma, USA

EDITORS

JEFFREY R. APPLEGATE Jr, DVM
Diplomate, American College of Zoological Medicine; Medical Director/Veterinarian, Nautilus Avian and Exotics Veterinary Specialists, Brick, New Jersey, USA; Adjunct Clinical Assistant Professor, Department of Clinical Sciences, North Carolina State University, College of Veterinary Medicine, Founding Member, Past President, Honey Bee Veterinary Consortium, Raleigh, North Carolina, USA

BRITTENY KYLE, DVM
Department of Population Medicine, Ontario Veterinary College, University of Guelph, Guelph, Ontario, Canada; Past President, Honey Bee Veterinary Consortium, Raleigh, North Carolina, USA

AUTHORS

JEFFREY R. APPLEGATE Jr, DVM
Diplomate, American College of Zoological Medicine; Medical Director/Veterinarian, Nautilus Avian and Exotics Veterinary Specialists, Brick, New Jersey, USA; Adjunct Clinical Assistant Professor, Department of Clinical Sciences, North Carolina State University, College of Veterinary Medicine, Founding Member, Past President, Honey Bee Veterinary Consortium, Raleigh, North Carolina, USA

RICARDO ANGUIANO-BAEZ, DVM, MSc
Adjunct Professor, National Autonomous University of Mexico, Mexico City, Mexico

PRIYADARSHINI CHAKRABARTI, PhD
Mississippi State University, Mississippi State, Mississippi, USA; Oregon State University, Corvallis, Oregon, USA

BROOKE DECKER, MS
State Apiculturist, Vermont Agency of Agriculture, Food and Markets, Montpelier, Vermont, USA

TRACY S. FARONE, BS, DVM
Professor of Biology, Grove City College, Grove City, Pennsylvania, USA

CYNTHIA M. FAUX, DVM, PhD
Diplomat, American College of Veterinary Internal Medicine - Large Animal; Professor, Veterinary Medicine, The University of Arizona College of Veterinary Medicine, Oro Valley, Arizona, USA

NATASHA GARCIA-ANDERSEN, BS
Fish and Wildlife Biologist, Department of Energy and Environment, Washington, DC, USA

ERNESTO GUZMAN-NOVOA, PhD
Professor and Head of the Honey Bee Research Centre, University of Guelph, School of Environmental Sciences, Guelph, Ontario, Canada

DON I. HOPKINS
North Carolina State Apiarist, Snow Camp, North Carolina, USA; North Carolina Department of Agriculture and Consumer Services, Plant Industry Division, Raleigh, North Carolina, USA

TERRY RYAN KANE, DVM, MS
A2 Bee Vet, Ann Arbor, Michigan, USA

JENNIFER J. KELLER
Apiculture Research Technician, Department of Entomology and Plant Pathology, North Carolina State University, Raleigh, North Carolina, USA

BRITTENY KYLE, DVM
Department of Population Medicine, Ontario Veterinary College, University of Guelph, Guelph, Ontario, Canada; Past President, Honey Bee Veterinary Consortium, Raleigh, North Carolina, USA

KATIE LEE, MS, PhD
Apiculture Extension Educator and Research Scientist, University of Minnesota, Saint Paul, Minnesota, USA

JENNIFER LUND, MS
State Apiarist, Maine Department of Agriculture, Conservation and Forestry, Augusta, Maine, USA

NURIA MORFIN, PhD
Research Associate, University of Guelph, School of Environmental Sciences, Guelph, Ontario, Canada

DEBORAH J.M. PASHO, DVM
Veterinarian, Huckleberry Farm Bee Services, Hartland, Vermont, USA; Vice President 2020-2021, Honey Bee Veterinary Consortium, Greensboro, North Carolina, USA

STEPHEN F. PERNAL, PhD
Research Scientist, Agriculture and Agri-Food Canada, Beaverlodge Research Farm, Beaverlodge, Alberta, Canada

TAMMY HORN POTTER, PhD
State Apiarist, Kentucky Department of Agriculture, Frankfort, Kentucky, USA

SAMUEL D. RAMSEY, PhD
Research Fellow, Agricultural Research Service, Bee Research Laboratory, United States Department of Agriculture, Beltsville, Maryland, USA; Director, Ramsey Research Foundation, Temple Hills, Maryland, USA; Doctor of Philosophy in Entomology, University of Maryland, Bachelor of Science in Entomology, Cornell University

MARY REED, BS
Chief Apiary Inspector, Texas Apiary Inspection Service, College Station, Texas, USA

RAMESH R. SAGILI, PhD
Oregon State University, Corvallis, Oregon, USA

KIM SKYRM, PhD
Chief Apiary Inspector, Massachusetts Department of Agricultural Resources, West Springfield, Massachusetts, USA

TANUSHREE TIWARI, PhD Candidate
Department of Biology, York University, Toronto, Ontario, Canada

JENNIFER M. TSURUDA, PhD
University of Tennessee - Knoxville, Knoxville, Tennessee, USA

DANIEL WYNS, BS
Field Specialist, Bee Informed Partnership, Academic Specialist, Michigan State University, University of Michigan, Lansing, Michigan, USA

AMRO ZAYED, PhD
Professor and York Research Chair in Genomics, Department of Biology, York University, Toronto, Ontario, Canada

Contents

Honey bees fulfill a critical role as the principal managed pollinator for modern agricultural ecosystems, necessary for the production of many of the world's food crops. The beekeeper must be a knowledgeable manager of bee health, apicultural production systems, and food safety practices. Veterinarians play a vital role in apiculture in supporting beekeepers to treat current and emerging diseases and pests.

Honey bees have evolved to use pollen, nectar, and water as their principal food sources. Their success is linked to the establishment of large colonies with one female reproductive member, 3 distinct social castes, a division of labor among workers, and genetically diverse subfamilies. Colonies also have the ability to recruit and communicate through complex mechanisms including dance language and pheromones. Pheromones produced by the queen maintain social order in the colony and ensure that she remains as the only female to lay eggs. Finally, honey bee colonies reproduce and disperse through a mechanism called swarming.

Infectious and parasitic diseases plague honey bees similarly to that of other food animal species. A complete understanding of each is necessary for a honey bee veterinarian to establish a strong veterinarian-client-patient relationship and make sound treatment recommendations. Control and management of these diseases is paramount to success of the colony and apiary operation. The following is not meant to be an end-all of information on each of the common honey bee diseases but more so a review and photo-documentation of each. A deeper understanding can be established through various other sources previously published and referenced in this document.

Honey bee colonies can be afflicted by serious conditions beyond infectious etiologies. Noninfectious conditions, such as starvation, laying worker colonies, and environmental dysregulation, can be as devastating as any disease. Improper hive monitoring and care often are the underlying causes of noninfectious conditions and each condition may be prevented by instituting best management practices.

 video content accompanies this article at http://www.vetfood. theclinics.com.

Honey bees are faced with many diseases, some more serious than others. Observing irregularities during routine hive inspection may indicate potential problems. Not all disorders are equally important; some are more detrimental and need immediate attention, whereas others may only need time to clear up. It is important to be observant to be able to recognize these diseases and differentiate between them so the correct treatment may be done in a timely manner when needed to maintain the health of the colony. Colonies need to be healthy to survive and prosper.

A 2017 US Food and Drug Administration mandate requiring veterinary oversight for medically important antibiotics used in agricultural animals, including honey bees (*Apis mellifera* L.) created a "new" animal requiring veterinary involvement. Many resources are available describing medical formulations of antibiotics and other drugs used in the treatment of various honey bee maladies. The goal of this article is to summarize this information in an up-to-date, practical way for the clinician. At the time of this writing, only 3 antibiotics are approved for use in honey bees and require veterinary prescriptions or veterinary feed directives.

Honey bee (*Apis mellifera*) health and hive transport are regulated by local apiary programs composed of apiary inspectors. Inspectors monitor and ensure the health of honey bees through field visits to apiaries where they inspect, identify, diagnose, and provide recommendations for the treatment of honey bee health issues. Laws and regulations pertaining to beekeeping and honey bee health are present in most states, territories, and provinces. Veterinarians are encouraged to establish a relationship with their local apiary inspector to further support beekeepers and the management of healthy honey bee colonies.

Honey bee veterinary medicine is a developing field in Canada and the United States. Veterinarians interested in working with honey bees should develop a comprehensive knowledge base on disease dynamics as it applies to the individual, colony, apiary, and broader honey bee populations. There are currently several governmental, academic, and industry organizations that are carrying out epidemiological-based surveys. Although honey bees face unique challenges in regard to biosecurity, the basic principles still apply. Veterinarians can use their expertise in the area of biosecurity to make improvements to current protocols within the apiary and beekeeping operations.

The honey bee *Apis mellifera* is a model organism for sociogenomics and one of the most important managed pollinators. High mortalities experienced by honey bee colonies over the past several decades are expected to have a substantive effect on crop pollination and global food security. These threats and the availability of a growing number of genomic resources for the honey bee have motivated research on how genetics and genomics can be practically applied to manage bee health. The authors review 3 such applications: (1) Certification of bee lineages using single-polymorphism markers; (2) breeding bees using marker-assisted selection; (3) diagnosing honey bee stressors using biomarkers.

Honey bees face a broad range of threats globally. Many of these threats originate outside of North America because honey bees are an introduced species. Invasive pests are among the most widely distributed, damaging, and economically costly honey bee hive associates. As international trade and travel continue at a rapid pace, the list of invasive apicultural pests likely will grow. Details of these organisms' life history relevant to management and eradication efforts are addressed. Methods and proposed methods of detection and management encountered abroad are discussed.

This article reviews how veterinarians can assist their apiarist clients in identifying hazards and risks to the apiary. Veterinarians can work with clients to navigate the various phases of disaster planning and response, as well as be a source of information on biosecurity and disease prevention. A summary of insurance programs applicable to apiarists is provided.

Euthanasia of animals is a cornerstone of veterinary medicine. Currently, no official criteria are set for the euthanasia or dispatch of a honey bee colony. Many methods are used around the world and vary with regards to technique, materials, volume of agent used, and timing. Each method described has its own level of effectiveness, safety, and humaneness. Although current, commonly used, methodologies may not meet the criteria of humane euthanasia, veterinarians can still apply the professional standard to other key aspects of the act of euthanasia.

VETERINARY CLINICS OF NORTH AMERICA: FOOD ANIMAL PRACTICE

SERIES OF RELATED INTEREST

Veterinary Clinics: Equine Practice
https://www.vetequine.theclinics.com/

Preface

Honey Bee Veterinary Medicine: A Developing Field

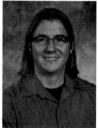

Jeffrey R. Applegate Jr, DVM, DACZM   Britteny Kyle, DVM
Editors

For generations, veterinarians have been at the forefront of disease management, herd health, and protecting against foreign animal disease. The Veterinarian's Oath, quoted from the American Veterinary Medical Association, states that a component of the veterinarian's responsibilities include: "…protection of animal health and welfare, the prevention and relief of animal suffering, the conservation of animal resources, the promotion of public health…." These concepts may be applied to all animals under veterinary care. Until recently, relative to the writing of this text, honey bees (*Apis mellifera*) have not been incorporated in the practice of veterinary medicine in North America. Now classified as food animals, honey bees require veterinary oversight to reduce antimicrobial resistance and prevent antibiotic residues in foods of animal origin.

Honey bees are fascinating animals that have a complex social structure and intricate communication strategies. Essential to modern agriculture, honey bees, driven by their natural behavior to collect nectar and pollen, are invaluable in the mass production of marketable fruits and vegetables. Along with native pollinators, honey bees fertilize almost three-quarters of the world's food crops intended for human consumption. These requirements place considerable demands on the apiculture industry. Beekeepers need to ensure sufficient numbers of strong colonies based on timing of crop blooming cycles rather than on honey bee natural foraging biology. Concurrently, in addition to commercial migratory stress, North American honey bee colonies are facing significant stressors, some of which include biosecurity challenges, nutritional deficits, diseases, parasites, and pests. Honey bee veterinary medicine involves a deeper understanding than simply when to administer antibiotics. A comprehensive understanding of commercial, sideline, and hobbyist apiculture is essential to be successful in this emerging field of veterinary medicine.

Veterinarians interested in working in the field of apiculture can utilize this text to build upon the framework of information provided in existing veterinary literature.

Vet Clin Food Anim 37 (2021) xiii–xiv
https://doi.org/10.1016/j.cvfa.2021.08.001
0749-0720/21/© 2021 Published by Elsevier Inc.

vetfood.theclinics.com

The need for veterinary care of honey bees may exist in scenarios as small as a single backyard hive to as complex as a commercial operation managing hundreds to thousands of hives across multiple locations. Information can be gleaned from this text for each scenario, developing a better understanding of the fundamentals of honey bee health, regulatory issues, commercial needs, and the application of veterinary medicine to honey bees.

Jeffrey R. Applegate Jr, DVM, DACZM
Nautilus Avian and Exotics Veterinary Specialists
1010 Falkenberg Road
Brick, NJ 08724, USA

Britteny Kyle, DVM
Department of Population Medicine
Ontario Veterinary College
50 Stone Road East
Guelph, Ontario N1G 2W1, Canada

E-mail addresses:
Drjeff@NAEVS.net (J.R. Applegate)
kyleb@uoguelph.ca (B. Kyle)

Introduction to Apiculture (*Apis mellifera*)

Stephen F. Pernal, PhD

KEYWORDS

• *Apis mellifera* • Beekeeping • Pollination

KEY POINTS

- Beekeeping has existed for thousands of years and has moved the Western honey bee, *Apis mellifera*, across the globe.
- Insect pollination is critical to world food production, and honey bees are the primary managed pollinators used in modern agriculture.
- Commercial beekeepers mange hundreds or thousands of colonies. They may move bees long distances to facilitate the pollination of high-value crops and produce honey that can be sold directly to consumers, with little or no processing.
- Beekeepers require veterinarians for access to disease-control products and to provide expert advice on managing pathogens and preventing antimicrobial resistance.

HISTORY

Honey has been a prized commodity since ancient times. Some of the oldest recorded evidence of honey collection is found in rock paintings from the Araña Caves in Spain, dating to approximately 13,000 BCE.[1] The practice of "hunting honey" from feral honey bees is still found in some indigenous societies today, whereby colonies are subdued with smoke and the nest is broken open to collect honeycombs.

A turning point in the domestication of honey bees (*Apis mellifera* L) was the understanding that a swarm could be enticed into an artificial nesting space specifically designed for the collection of honey and beeswax. Evidence of ancient beekeeping practices date to at least 2400 BCE, as shown in a stone bas-relief in the sun temple of Niuserre on the bank of the Nile River, where honey is being harvested and placed into containers.[2] Ancient Egyptian, Greek, and Roman societies all record keeping bees for the collection of honey, wax, and propolis, with the earliest forms of artificial hives made from hollow logs, wooden boxes, clay pots, or woven baskets. The oldest large-scale apiary ever unearthed, from the ancient town of Tel Rehov in Israel, contains beehives made from clay cylinders dating from 1000 to 900 BCE.[3] Honey was clearly prized as the only sweetener available to early African, Middle Eastern, and

Agriculture and Agri-Food Canada, Beaverlodge Research Farm, P.O. Box 29, Beaverlodge, Alberta T0H 0C0, Canada
E-mail address: Steve.Pernal@Canada.ca

European societies. Medieval Europe saw increases in the domestication of honey bees with greater demand for honey and wax, with the Christian religion being a major consumer of beeswax candles.[1,2,4] Over time, Europe introduced many innovations in terms of beekeeping and an improved understanding of bee biology.[5]

Honey bees were moved with humans on most major migrations and were brought to the New World in the early 1600s when European settlers introduced *A mellifera* to North America and Australasia.[1,6] Although advances continued in Europe with beekeeping equipment featuring side-opening hives, modern commercial beekeeping owes its existence to the development of the movable wooden frame hive that was developed in America by the Rev. Lorenzo L. Langstroth in 1851[7] (**Fig. 1**). The Langstroth hive was designed around the idea of "bee space", defined as spaces just large enough for bees to pass through, thereby limiting where they could build comb. This permitted beekeepers to have hives in which bees built comb in wooden frames that could be easily removed to assess hive health and productivity or to harvest honey. In 1865, the first honey extractor was developed,[1] allowing the centrifugal removal of honey from comb, thereby eliminating the former need to press and destroy the comb for harvest.

Today, beekeeping is a worldwide endeavor with *A mellifera* found in all but the extreme polar regions of the world. Across the globe, more than 90 million colonies are kept for the production of hive products and pollination.[8]

DISCUSSION
Importance of Bees

There are more than 20,000 named species of bees in the world[9] that play diverse functions in their respective ecosystems. These roles include pollination in wild and managed landscapes, providing food for animals, and involvement in the coevolution of plants. The seeds and fruits resulting from pollinating activities are critical to the livelihood, survival, and reproduction of countless animal species. More than 87% of wild plants require animals to pollinate their flowers in temperate and tropical ecosystems.[10] Although these pollinators may include birds, bats, mice, and lemurs, most are pollinated by insects. Among the numerous insects that visit flowers, bee species are the predominant pollinators.

Although the role of bees is often misunderstood, the most economically important role of bees is not the production of honey, but the pollination of crops. The reliance of humans on animal-pollinated crops demonstrates the value of services provided by

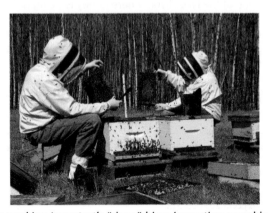

Fig. 1. Beekeepers working Langstroth "deep" hives inspecting movable frames.

pollinators to ecosystems: 76% of the world's leading food crops show increased fruit or seed set with animal pollination, comprising about 35% of the volume of the food produced.[11] The value of this pollination benefit is estimated at €153 billion (~$182 billion [USD]) annually, or 9.5% of the world value of commercial agricultural production used for food.[12] Honey bees (*A mellifera*) are the principal managed pollinator of most crops.[11,13] To enable this effort, growers set up contracts with beekeepers who move their colonies into a crop as it comes into bloom. Examples of major crops requiring honey bee pollination in North America include almond, blueberry, apple, cherry, cranberry, melon, plum/prune, avocado, pear, cucumber, sunflower, raspberry, alfalfa seed, and hybrid canola seed. The sheer demand for pollination services is evidenced by the fact that approximately 60% to 70% of all US honey bees are moved to California each year to meet the needs of almond growers.[14] Despite the worldwide increase in the number of managed honey bees colonies over the last half-century (~45%), this growth has not been able to keep pace with the increased demand for insect-dependent pollinated crops over the same time period (>300%).[15] As wild (non-*Apis*) bee pollinators also make smaller, although important, contributions to crop pollination,[13,16] the future for crop production may be that of an integrated crop pollination model in which wild and managed bee species are used in concert to pollinate crops. Such an approach requires farm management practices that support and protect native pollinator populations, including augmenting and preserving natural habitat in agricultural landscapes, using appropriate pesticide stewardship, and developing improved horticultural practices.[17] As the area of pollinator-dependent crops continues to expand while threats to honey bee health do not diminish, solutions to meet crop pollination deficits are likely to become an increasing priority for the future of agriculture.

The Beekeeper

A typical beekeeper or beekeeping operation is difficult to generalize, as practices vary among regions and countries. Most beekeepers are hobbyist or small scale, whereas a minority are large commercial beekeepers who derive their living exclusively from bees. For example, of the ~120,000 beekeepers in the United States, 60% of all honey is produced by about 1600 commercial beekeepers, categorized as operating greater than 300 colonies each.[18] In the summer of 2019, the United States had in excess of 3 million honey bee colonies,[19] which produced 71,000 tons of raw honey valued at $309 million (USD).[20] Annual income received by US beekeepers for pollination services is estimated at $435 million (USD),[21] whereas the contribution of honey bee pollination to the value of US crops exceeds $19 billion (USD).[22,23] Similarities exist in Canada, with a population of approximately 12,000 beekeepers and 747,000 colonies that produced 38,000 tons of honey valued at $209 million (CAD) in 2020.[24] This value is a fraction of the $4 to $5.5 billion (CAD) economic contribution that honey bee pollination provides to the value of Canadian agricultural crops.[25]

The natural activities of honey bee colonies are principally divided between balancing the need to reproduce at the colony level (swarming) and storing enough honey to survive over winter months. In temperate climates, a beekeeping year follows an annual cycle of growth, which begins in the spring when pollen is available, leading to rapid expansion of the nest in which 30,000 brood cells can be produced by late spring to early summer.[26] Typically at this point in the season, colonies may have gaps in brood rearing owing to increasing queen and drone rearing, in anticipation of swarming. From mid to late spring until the fall, the colony focusss on establishing a sufficient supply of honey to survive the winter. Depending on regional conditions, one or several nectar flows may exist in which sufficient flora bloom to enable colonies to collect large amounts of nectar, then process and store it as honey to meet their short-term and future energetic requirements. During the fall, brood rearing dwindles and long-lived bees that will survive the winter months are produced.

Commercial beekeepers are the managers of insect livestock and must work with their hives to produce honey and pollinate crops. They must use their knowledge of honey bee biology to prevent colonies form naturally swarming, often by splitting colonies or providing them with more space, in order for them to be of the desired size and strength for honey production or pollinating activities. Beekeepers must also purchase, or select and breed, new queens in order to control stock genetics, and to counter the effects of uncontrolled mating of naturally produced virgin queens in their operation. Uncontrolled swarming of colonies also leads to the loss of bees to unknown locations, smaller net remaining parent colonies, and long broodless periods as virgin queens mate with unselected drones and then start egg laying. Beekeepers also aggressively harvest the honey that bees have produced throughout the spring and summer, effectively robbing them of the resource they need to survive the winter. Consequently, beekeepers must feed colonies large quantities of sugar syrup during fall periods in order to prevent colonies starving over winter. In northern temperate climates, the gross weight of colonies being prepared for winter is recommended to be as much as 63 to 73 kg,[27] with much of this weight being beekeeper-fed sugar syrup and stored honey.

Although honey bee colonies would naturally be stationary, beekeepers frequently move their colonies to exploit nectar sources or to pollinate crops. Such migratory beekeeping may occur over long distances, often several hundred or even thousands of kilometers. Moving colonies can be stressful for bees and often requires regulatory inspections before or after the bees are moved across regional boundaries, to prevent the spread of unwanted diseases or pests.

A beekeeper is responsible for assessing the health of their hives, checking for mite infestations, and maintaining detailed records of queen status, colony state, treatments applied, and honey production. Beekeepers in most parts of the world work closely with veterinarians for the application of treatments to hives, particularly if antibiotics are required for the treatment of brood diseases, such as American and European foulbrood North America. In most countries, commercial beekeepers also follow stringent biosecurity standards and food safety regulations, the latter requiring fully traceable and inspected honey production establishments.[28,29]

Beekeepers possess a broad array of skills to manage an insect pollinator that plays such a large role in world food production. In many instances, they must manage against the natural tendencies of honey bee colonies and move hives that would naturally be stationary. Furthermore, they must be a good steward of this insect's health, control stock genetics and produce one of the few food products that is sold to consumers requiring little or no processing, meeting all necessary guidelines for safe food production. Dedication, knowledge, and a tolerance to venomous stings are required to succeed in this unique profession, to which the world owes so much.

SUMMARY

The practice of keeping bees by humans has occurred over thousands of years. Honey bees are among the most highly evolved social insects that live in communal societies. Humans have been able to domesticate them through the use of artificial nest structures, which allow for manipulation and transport. Beekeepers play an extremely important role in apiculture, as they are able to manipulate honey bees to meet global pollination needs of modern agriculture. Beekeepers need to work closely with veterinarians to ensure optimal colony health, the use of proper treatments, and for area-management strategies for emerging diseases and pests. Veterinarians also have an important role in monitoring for disease outbreaks and antibiotic-resistant pathogens. Finally, veterinarians are a resource to support beekeepers, provincial and state apiculturalists, and extension agents, for the benefit of apiculture and agriculture as a whole.

CLINICS CARE POINTS

- Most beekeepers are hobbyists or part-time beekeepers operating a small number of colonies. There are far fewer commercial beekeepers, who operate far greater numbers of colonies, produce most honey sold for consumers, and are responsible for all managed crop pollination.

- Veterinarians will have hobbyist, part-time, and commercial beekeeping clients with widely diverging resources and needs. Clients will be concerned with timely and appropriate access to disease control products, and the management of more virulent or treatment-resistant pathogens and pests.

- Veterinarians should endeavor to have a thorough understanding of honey bee biology and commercial beekeeping practices should they wish to engage beekeeping clients.

DISCLOSURE

The author has nothing to disclose.

REFERENCES

1. Crane E. The world history of beekeeping and honey hunting. London: Gerald Duckworth & Co; 1999.
2. Crane E. The archaeology of beekeeping. 1st edition. London: Gerald Duckworth & Co; 1983.
3. Bloch G, Francoy TM, Wachtel I, et al. Industrial apiculture in the Jordan Valley during biblical times with Anatolian honeybees. Proc Natl Acad Sci U S A 2010;107:11240–4.
4. Free JB. Bees and mankind. London: George Allen & Unwin; 1982.
5. More D. The bee book: the history and natural history of the honeybee. New York: Universe Books; 1976.
6. Smith DA. The first honeybees in America. Bee World 1977;58:56.
7. Dadant CC. Beekeeping equipment. In: Graham JM, editor. The hive and the honey bee. Hamilton, IL: Dadant and Sons; 1992. p. 537–73.
8. FAOSTAT. Food and Agriculture Organization of the United Nations. Livestock Primary. Available at: http://www.fao.org/faostat/en/#data/QL. Accessed December 31, 2020.
9. Orr MC, Hughes AC, Chesters D, et al. Global patterns and drivers of bee distribution. Curr Biol 2021;31:451–8.
10. Ollerton J, Winfree R, Tarrant S. How many flowering plants are pollinated by animals? Oikos 2011;120:321–6.
11. Klein A-M, Vaissière BE, Cane JH, et al. Importance of pollinators in changing landscapes for world crops. Proc R Soc B 2007;274:303–13.

12. Gallai N, Salles J-M, Settele J, et al. Economic valuation of the vulnerability of world agriculture confronted with pollinator decline. Ecol Econ 2009;68:810–21.

13. Garibaldi L, Steffan-Dewenter I, Winfree E, et al. Wild pollinators enhance fruit set of crops regardless of honey bee abundance. Science 2013;339:1608–11.

14. Ferrier P, Rucker RR, Thurman WN, et al. Economic effects and responses to changes in honey bee health. Washington, DC: U.S. Department of Agriculture, Economic Research Service; 2018. Economic Research Report ERR-246, Available at: https://www.ers.usda.gov/publications/pub-details/?pubid=88116.

15. Aizen MA, Harder LD. The global stock of domesticated honey bees is growing slower than agricultural demand for pollination. Curr Biol 2009;19:915–8.

16. Winfree R, Gross BJ, Kremen C. Valuing pollination services to agriculture. Ecol Econ 2011;71:80–8.

17. Isaacs R, Williams N, Ellis J, et al. Integrated crop pollination: combining strategies to ensure stable and sustainable yields of pollination-dependent crops. Basic Appl Ecol 2017;22:44–60.

18. Agricultural Marketing Resource Center. Bees. Available at: https://www.agmrc.org/commodities-products/livestock/bees-profile. Accessed December 31, 2020.

19. Honey Bee Colonies. United States Department of Agriculture, National Agricultural Statistics Service. 2020. Available at: https://downloads.usda.library.cornell.edu/usda-esmis/files/rn301137d/nc5819380/t148g6070/hcny0820.pdf. Accessed December 31, 2020.

20. Honey. United States Department of Agriculture, National Agricultural Statistics Service. 2020. Available at: https://downloads.usda.library.cornell.edu/usda-esmis/files/hd76s004z/v979vm595/dn39xk32q/hony0320.pdf. Accessed December 31, 2020.

21. Costs of Pollination. United States Department of agriculture, National agricultural Statistics service 2017. Available at: https://downloads.usda.library.cornell.edu/usda-esmis/files/d504rk335/ht24wn48h/zg64tp76q/CostPoll-12-21-2017.pdf. Accessed December 31, 2020.

22. Morse RA, Calderone NW. The value of honey bees as pollinators of U.S. crops in 2000. Bee Cult 2000;128:1–15.

23. Calderone NW. Insect pollinated crops, insect pollinators and US agriculture: trend analysis of aggregate data for the period 1992–2009. PLoS One 2012;7(5):e37235.

24. Statistics Canada. Table 32-10-0353-01 production and value of honey. Available at: https://doi.org/10.25318/3210035301-eng. Accessed December 31, 2020.

25. Mukezangango J, Page S. Statistical overview of the Canadian honey and bee industry and the economic contribution of honey bee pollination 2016. AAFC No.12715E 2017. Available at: https://www.agr.gc.ca/resources/prod/doc/pdf/honey_2016-eng.pdf. Accessed December 31, 2020.

26. Seeley TD. Honeybee ecology: a study of adaptation in social life. Princeton (NJ): Princeton University Press; 1985.

27. Gruszka J, editor. Beekeeping in Western Canada. Edmonton, AB: Alberta Agriculture, Food and Rural Development; 1998.

28. Canadian Food Inspection Agency. National Bee Farm-Level Biosecurity Standard. Available at: https://www.inspection.gc.ca/animal-health/terrestrial-animals/biosecurity/standards-and-principles/bee-industry/eng/1365794112591/1365794221593?chap=0. Accessed December 31, 2020.

29. Canadian Food Inspection Agency. Safe food for Canadians regulations. Available at: https://laws-lois.justice.gc.ca/eng/regulations/SOR-2018-108/FullText.html. Accessed December 31, 2020.

The Social Life of Honey Bees

Stephen F. Pernal, PhD

KEYWORDS

- *Apis mellifera* • Sociality • Dance language • Pheromones • Swarming

KEY POINTS

- Honey bees live in highly evolved social societies with distinct castes, a division of labor among workers, and overlapping generations.
- Honey bees communicate through dance language and chemical signals (pheromones) for recruitment to food sources and to maintain social hierarchy.
- Populous colonies naturally reproduce by swarming. Beekeepers manage colony populations to reduce this propensity, as swarming reduces within-season productivity.

INTRODUCTION

Honey bees have evolved to be among the most complex of all insect societies in which there is a division into morphologically distinct social castes and a high degree of social cooperation and efficiency among nestmates. Honey bee colonies also normally have only one female reproductive member, the queen, who is highly promiscuous and mates with numerous males (drones) to maximize the genetic diversity of the colony. Although honey bees live in a dark hive, they are able to communicate in several fascinating ways, including well-characterized "dances," which tell nestmates where to exploit food resources, as well as numerous chemical signals that allow the queen to maintain control over the colony, enable larvae to express hunger to nurses, and assist workers in orientation. All these forms of communication allow honey bees to live in a highly integrated society, promoting the fitness and survival of the colony as a whole.

DISCUSSION
Members of a Colony

Honey bees have three castes in their society: workers, drones, and queens (**Fig. 1**). Workers and queens are female and develop from fertilized eggs, whereas drones are male and develop from unfertilized eggs, in a reproductive system known as

Agriculture and Agri-Food Canada, Beaverlodge Research Farm, P.O. Box 29, Beaverlodge, Alberta, Canada, T0H 0C0
E-mail address: Steve.Pernal@Canada.ca

Vet Clin Food Anim 37 (2021) 387–400
https://doi.org/10.1016/j.cvfa.2021.06.012
0749-0720/21/Crown Copyright © 2021 Published by Elsevier Inc. All rights reserved.
vetfood.theclinics.com

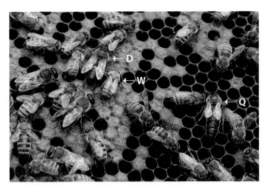

Fig. 1. Three honey bee castes on a frame, examples of D, drone; W, worker; Q, queen.

haplodiploidy. There is normally one queen in a honey bee nest, several thousand workers, and a smaller proportion of drones. Unless indicated, information in this section is drawn from previous reviews of bee development and biology.[1,2]

Honey bees are holometabolous insects, undergoing a complete metamorphosis having egg, larval, pupal, and adult stages. The immature stages (egg, larva, and pupa) are collectively known as brood and are maintained in the center of the nest at approximately 35°C (95°F) via the heat produced from adult bees. All life stage development occurs within cells in the wax comb. Eggs and larvae develop in uncapped brood cells; however, prepupal and pupal stages develop after cells are sealed by the workers. The queen lays an egg at the base of each cell in an upright position, hatching as a larva after 3 days. Diploid female larvae that are less than 3 days old are considered to be totipotent, having the capacity to develop into either queens or workers. Fertilized eggs that are destined to become queens are laid in a special cell, known as a queen cup, which is a vertically oriented, cup-shaped cell found on the face or bottom edge of the comb surface. When mature, queen cups become elongated by the workers and capped (**Fig. 2**). The differentiation of a young female larva into a queen or worker depends on the quantity and composition of the diet that is fed to the larva by young adult workers, known as "nurse bees". Queen larvae are fed "royal jelly" for their entire development, consisting of secretions from the

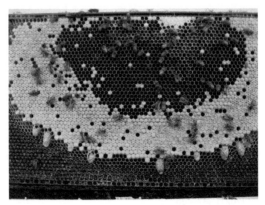

Fig. 2. Elongated, peanut-shaped queen cells developing along the periphery of the brood area.

hypopharyngeal and mandibular glands of nurse bees. These secretions contain a higher proportion of mandibular gland components and sugars compared with worker food. Worker larvae are fed a diet known as "brood food", consisting of high proportions of hypopharyngeal gland components during their first few days of development, with honey and pollen being introduced during the latter days of development. Drone larvae receive a diet similar to workers, although a larger quantity owing to their larger body size. Average developmental times from egg to adult emergence vary slightly, but are generally recognized as 16 days for queens, 21 days for workers, and 24 days for drones.

Each adult caste in a honey bee colony has a specialized role. Queen bees are normally the sole female reproductive member in honey bee colonies. When preparing to swarm or replace a dead or failing queen, a colony will rear many virgin queens. Approximately 3 days after emergence, a virgin queen will embark on a series of mating flights in which she searches for drone congregation areas where drones from many different colonies will be found. Honey bee queens are considered hyperpolyandrous, being promiscuous and mating with a large number of drones, creating several patrilines or subfamilies of workers related to each other in the hive. Although estimates of queen mating frequency have previously indicated an average of approximately 12 drone matings per queen,[3] the presence of recently discovered, rare "royal patrilines" suggests that in excess of 50 drones may actually mate per queen.[4] Queen polyandry is recognized as a strategy to confer greater fitness and productivity for the colony as a whole,[5] as well as increased resistance to disease.[6] Drones deposit sperm in the queen where it is stored in her spermatheca and used continuously over her lifetime, eliminating the need for her to leave the nest again for mating purposes. Queens live between 1 and 3 years and lay approximately 1500 eggs per day during summer months and in excess of 500,000 in their lifetime.[7]

Worker bees comprise most of a colony's total population, which may peak at 40,000 to 60,000 during summer months. To defend their colony at the cost of their own life, workers have a barbed sting attached to a poison sack and are also equipped with other specialized features, such as branched hairs across their body for the collection of pollen, pollen baskets (corbiculae) on the tibia of their hind legs to carry pollen back to the hive, and a honey stomach to transport nectar. Workers are responsible for most in-hive tasks and progress through a predictable age-related division of labor, known as *temporal polyethism*. This progression starts with cell cleaning after a new worker emerges and then moves onto feeding brood, capping brood, trimming cappings, attending the queen, grooming, feeding nestmates, ventilating the hive, building comb, removing debris, receiving nectar from foragers, concentrating nectar, storing nectar, capping honey, packing pollen, guarding the entrance of the nest, and finally, foraging[7] (**Fig. 3**). As such, younger workers spend their time inside the nest, whereas older workers perform the more hazardous duties of food collection. During the summer, workers live up to 6 weeks[8]; however, over winter months winter workers may live in excess of 140 days,[9] with some records indicating survivorship beyond 300 days.[10,11]

Drones develop from larger cells than workers, with these being built near the periphery of the nest or where patches of worker comb have been damaged. Colonies produce drones during spring and summer months when virgin queens are likely to be produced. Drones are approximately twice the size of workers, with larger eyes and sensitive antennae to assist in locating drone congregation areas and queens in flight. Drones lack pollen baskets and have small tongues and mandibles. The principal contribution drones make to the well-being of the hive is passing on genetic material by mating with queens.[12] From 5 to 8 days after emerging as an adult, drones will

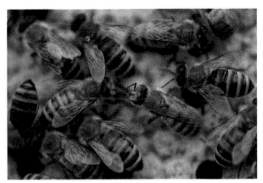

Fig. 3. One of the many behavioral tasks of workers: sharing food with nest mates through trophallaxis.

take short orientation flights and will embark on actual mating flights within 10 days. Mating flights are typically within 15 to 40 m of the ground in an area of 20 to 200 m diameter.[13] When a queen enters the drone congregation area she is followed by a comet of drones; a successful drone will mount her from above, grasping her with his legs; however, the queen must voluntarily open her sting chamber for copulation to take place.[14] After copulation, drones become paralyzed, fall to the ground, and die. As summer draws to a close, drones remaining in the colony are ejected by the workers, because they will consume colony stores and will not contribute to the fitness of the colony.

Sociality

Bee species in general may exhibit three levels of social organization: solitary, presocial, and eusocial.[15,16] The classification among these three levels of organization depends on the degree to which species display the following social requirements: (1) cooperative brood care, whereby multiple members of the same species rear immatures not of their own; (2) reproductive division of labor, in which one, or a few individuals, reproduce, whereas the others rear immatures and perform nest-related tasks; and (3) overlapping generations, whereby multiple generations perform tasks in the nest together. Most bee species in the world are strictly solitary in which a single female emerges from her nest as an adult, mates, locates a new nest, provisions it with pollen and nectar, lays eggs, seals the cells, and then leaves before the offspring emerge. The offspring eat the provisions and later emerge to repeat the cycle. Presocial bees are ones that exhibit any of the three social requirements, but not all, and can be further classified into those that are subsocial and parasocial.

Eusocial bees, such as *Apis mellifera*, exhibit all three social requirements. These bees have a reproductive division of labor, in that some females are responsible for egg laying, whereas others are responsible for nonreproductive labor tasks. Only the queen in a honey bee colony is mated and can lay fertilized eggs. The nonreproductive workers feed and care for the brood, defend the hive, maintain its infrastructure, and forage. Honey bees also have cooperative brood care in which the brood is fed by adults and workers that do not care for their own offspring, but of that of the queen. In addition, honey bees have overlapping generations whereby at least two generations, queen and worker, are mature at the same time with workers contributing to the labor of the colony. As queens and workers are not structurally similar and queens are not capable of living alone, honey bees are considered to be highly eusocial, in contrast to queens from primitively eusocial species, such as bumble bees, which can survive by themselves.

Eusocial organisms, such as honey bees, are subject to both the benefits and costs of group living.[17] Large social groups can serve as defense against predation, allow advantages against competitors, and permit more efficient collection of food. Honey bees also exhibit social immunity, whereby social behaviors such as hygienic removal of brood, production of antibacterial resin (propolis), social grooming, and fever can be used to fight against diseases and parasites.[18,19] There can also be costs to living in social groups, such as increased competition for resources between individuals, increased disease and parasite transmission, and simplified detection of the nest by predators; ultimately these are offset by fitness advantages.

Dance Language

Workers returning to the hive after a foraging trip may communicate the location of a profitable food source using what is known as "dance language." Descriptions are drawn from extensive reviews on this topic.[1,15,20–23]

The round dance is the simpler of the two forms of dance communication. This dance does not encode specific distance or direction information; instead it conveys to foragers that a high-quality food resource is within 15 m of the hive. During this dance, the dancing worker shares nectar with nestmates while they follow and antennate her. The dancer makes repeated small circles on the comb of the hive, reversing her course every 1 or 2 revolutions, for only a few seconds or up to several minutes

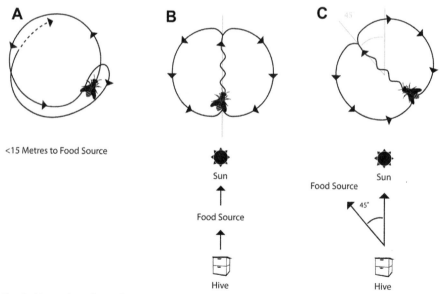

Fig. 4. Honey bee dance language. (*A*) Round dances used to communicate food sources less than 15 m from the hive. (*B* and *C*) Waggle dances used to communicate a food source greater than 100 m from the hive. In (*B*) the food source is directly toward the sun, with the dancer preforming its waggle run directly up the comb. In (*C*) the food source is 45° to the left of the sun, with the dancer orienting its waggle run the same angle to the left of vertical on the comb. The duration of waggling and buzzing during the straight run, as well as overall dance tempo, are the primary cues encoding the distance of the resource from the hive.

(**Fig. 4**A). The profitability of a food reward is communicated in the round dance, whereby the vigor and length of dances increase with nectars having greater sugar concentration. Recruits fly in widening circles from the nest and locate the food source using floral cues detected from the dancer. Pollen foragers also perform the round dance. Attending workers are quickly recruited to the location of the flowers bearing the same odor as that produced by the pollen.[24]

The waggle dance communicates specific information about the distance and direction of a food source in relation to the position of the hive, as well as the food source quality. Waggle dances are normally performed only at distances of 100 m or more, with bees performing a transition dance, which is a gradual change between the round and waggle dance, at distances between 25 and 100 m. The returning forager dances a figure-eight pattern on the comb, with the middle portion of the dance being termed the *straight run* (see **Fig. 4**B). During the straight run, the worker travels ahead for a short distance shaking her body vigorously from side to side at a rate of 13 to 15 times per second, with a buzzing sound also being given off. At the end of each straight run, the forager makes a semicircular arc back to the starting point, to do another straight run and then a turn in the opposite direction. Similar to the round dance, the dancing forager will stop to exchange food with nearby workers who typically surround the dancer in a tight retinue with extended antennae. The orientation of the straight run indicates the direction of the food source, using the sun as a reference or compass, effectively transposing the horizontal direction to a solar angle. In terms of direction, when viewing the comb, the sun is considered to be on the top. For example, if the straight run is 45° to the left of top, the resource is located 45° to the left of the sun (see **Fig 4**C). For distance, several features are evaluated by workers to determine how far the resource is away; however, the two most indicative features are the duration of waggling and buzzing during the straight run and the overall dance tempo. The tempo of dances will slow with greater distance, and the time in the straight run increases for a resource further away. Notably, foragers do not communicate absolute distance but the amount of energy expended to fly there. The same components of the dance that indicate distance also provide information about the quality of the resource collected. In particular, the dance characteristics that code for quality or profitability include the lateral extent of waggling, the total number of dance cycles, and the intensity of the buzzing vibrations.

Other vibratory signals and dances occur in the hive, with better and lesser-known functions.[25–27] One example is the dorsoventral abdominal vibration (DVAV), or vibration dance, which differs from the round and waggle dances in tuning the daily and seasonal foraging patterns to varying resource supplies in the environment. Workers vibrate their bodies, particularly their abdomens, in a dorsoventral plane, typically while in contact with another bee. Vibration dances tend to increase at times of the day and season when the colony needs to be activated for higher levels of foraging, with these dances functioning to concentrate potential recruits into the area where waggle dances are being performed. Other researchers suggest that DVAV signals may have additional functions beyond foraging activation, with the amplitude of the signal indicating this switching of purpose; vibration signals also frequently precede and follow primary swarms.[28]

Chemical Communication

Honey bees also communicate through their chemical language, using pheromones. Pheromones are chemical signals that have evolved for communication between members of the same species.[29] Honey bee queens, workers, drones, and larvae all have exocrine glands to secrete chemicals that remain as liquids or evaporate. These chemicals are perceived through receptors and transferred through antennal contact, food exchange (trophallaxis), grooming, or marking of resources.[30]

The honey bee queen is the principal regulator of colony function. To accomplish this, she disseminates a variety of compounds that are produced by different glands and are emitted as a complex chemical blend, often referred to as the *queen signal*. The queen signal acts mainly as a primer pheromone, causing physiologic and behavioral modifications in workers that create a social hierarchy in the colony and maintain homeostasis. The main component of the queen signal is known as *queen mandibular pheromone* (QMP), which was discovered to be a 5-component blend of compounds secreted by the mandibular gland.[31] These compounds were found to elicit formation of the retinue response in workers, normally seen as the "court" of workers surrounding the queen in a hive[32] (**Fig. 5**). In the years since the discovery of the 5-component blend of QMP, four additional components were identified, which, when added to QMP, more fully characterize the chemical activity seen in bioassays using extracts of actual queen mandibular glands. This 9-component blend was termed *queen retinue pheromone* (QRP)[33] and is the most complex single pheromone known for inducing behavior in any organism.[34]

The substances that comprise queen pheromones ensure the queen remains the only reproductive member in the colony by suppressing ovary development in workers and preventing new queen rearing.[35] Pheromone components also stimulate workers to forage and rear brood,[36] build comb,[37] clean cells, and guard the nest[38] and are important in worker recognition of the queen.[1] When queens are old and produce a weak pheromonal signal, or die leaving the colony with none, workers will quickly produce new queens from young worker brood within 12 to 24 hours.[1] If a new queen does not develop, some workers will develop their own ovaries and lay unfertilized (drone) eggs[39,40]; if a beekeeper cannot artificially introduce a new queen to a colony incapable of producing their own, the colony will dwindle and die.

Queen pheromones are primarily disseminated by contact.[33] In the retinue, young workers attend the queen, licking and touching her with their antennae, removing pheromone from her body and often retaining sufficient quantities to become attractive to other workers after leaving the queen.[41] In a large, growing colony, the concentration of pheromone is lessened particularly toward the periphery of the nest,[42] decreasing the queen's ability to inhibit queen rearing and prevent swarming. When colonies do swarm, queen pheromones serve as an attractant for bees to cluster with their queen[43] and serve to attract drones for mating.

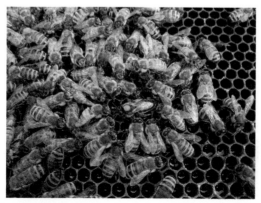

Fig. 5. A retinue of workers surrounding the queen in the hive. The queen is marked with a green paint dot on her thorax to facilitate her being found by the beekeeper.

Aside from the queen, worker bees also produce several pheromones. The pheromone produced by the Nasonov gland is composed of seven volatile chemicals and elicits orientation and recruitment of workers.[44] Workers expose their Nasonov gland, located on the upper posterior of the abdomen between the sixth and seventh tergites, and disperse the odor by fanning their wings (**Fig. 6**). Scenting with the Nasonov gland occurs at the nest entrance particularly after a colony is disturbed, when foraging for water, or to mark foraging sites with little natural odor.[29,45,46] Nasonov compounds are also important for orientation during swarming, including clustering after swarming, and to orient to new nesting sites.[29] Other studies suggest a role of Nasonov pheromone within the hive whereby workers expose their Nasonov gland when choosing young larvae to rear as new queens, to attract other workers toward the selected cell.[47]

Worker bees also secrete pheromones from their tarsi, or feet, called *footprint* pheromones, which is believed to originate from the tarsal (Arnhart) glands.[48] This pheromone is suggested to serve a secondary role in marking the hive entrance and at food sources; it is deposited on the colony entrance by alighting workers and on visited flowers, further enhancing the attractiveness of the Nasonov pheromone.[49] Footprint pheromone is hypothesized to act as a proximity signal at short distances, whereas Nasonov pheromone is more broadly attractive, having volatile components being perceived at greater distances.[50]

Workers additionally produce alarm pheromones, primarily secreted by the Koschevnikov gland and by the glandular areas of the sting sheaths,[38] as well as from the mandibular glands. As such, there are two main groups of substances with alarm effects: the sting apparatus alarm pheromone, which has as a main component isopentyl acetate (IPA),[51,52] and the mandibular gland alarm pheromone, composed only of 2-heptanone.[53] Both substances elicit defensive behavior against threats at the hive entrance; however, those produced by the sting apparatus elicit much greater biological activity for recruiting bees and inducing stinging behavior, suggesting that the two glandular substances have different functional roles even if both are capable of evoking defensive responses.[54]

Defensive behavior is one of the first out-of-nest nest tasks performed by worker bees. Workers typically disperse the alarm pheromone by exposing their sting apparatus and fanning vigorously with their wings.[29] When this activity occurs by a guard bee at the hive entrance, other workers sensing the alarm pheromone will join her

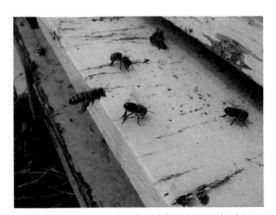

Fig. 6. Workers exposing their Nasonov gland and fanning at the hive entrance. The glands are located on the upper posterior surface of the abdomen.

and will have a low threshold to sting anything that is perceived to be a threat to the colony, particularly those with contrasting patterns and movements. When an animal is stung, the barbs of a worker bee sting will remain in its flesh resulting in the sting and poison sac being torn from the bee as it attempts to fly away. The poison sac is coated in alarm pheromone and marks the spot to be attacked by other bees.

Honey bee races that differ in the intensity of defensive behavior can show differences in the amount and composition of alarm pheromones. Notably, Africanized bees, *A mellifera scutella*, often coined "killer bees" by the general public, have been found to contain higher levels for 9 of 12 sting-derived alarm pheromone components compared with European races of bees and twice as much IPA.[55] In addition, derivatives of IPA found specifically in the alarm pheromone of Africanized bees, in combination with existing pheromone components, provide for synergistic recruitment of workers.[56] These factors contribute to a much lower threshold of response by Africanized honey bees and much greater intensity of defensive response.

Honey bee larvae produce a mixture of compounds that function to regulate colony growth and worker maturation. These compounds are collectively known as brood pheromone, which is a blend of 10 fatty acid methyl and ethyl esters.[57] Brood pheromone is secreted by the salivary glands and varies in function with the caste and age of the larvae. For example, four of the esters act as cues for workers to initiate larval cell capping,[58] whereas other components increase the activity of the worker hypopharyngeal glands for the production of brood food.[59] During queen rearing, other pheromone components increase the acceptance of queen cell cups, the amount of royal jelly fed, and the weight of the resulting queen larvae.[60] Colonies treated with artificial brood pheromone also rear more brood and adults than control colonies and have increased protein consumption.[61] Similarly-treated colonies also increase their ratio of pollen to nonpollen food collectors and the size of the pollen loads collected.[62] In addition, brood pheromone-treated colonies have better-fed queens, which lay more eggs, and workers that spend more time cleaning cells and tending brood.[62,63] Finally, brood pheromone components work in conjunction with QMP and the larval-derived volatile known as E-β-ocimene,[64] to inhibit worker ovarian development, likely by lowering juvenile hormone titers.[65]

Colony Reproduction

Honey bee colonies reproduce by swarming, a process that is composed of an array of collective behaviors that have evolved to enhance reproductive success by dividing a populous colony into new units. It is an epic event in which most workers and a queen leave the nest to locate a new site to live, filling the air with thousands of bees searching for their queen and somewhere to cluster. In temperate climates, swarming normally occurs during midspring and early summer months. During this time, a colony's population will expand until it is too large for its maternal nest, at which point the colony will proceed to divide.[66] Several factors are known to influence the probability of swarming, including increases in colony size, brood nest congestion, high proportions of young workers, decreased transmission of queen pheromones, and the availability of nectar and pollen in the environment.[1] Preparations for swarming occur 2 to 4 weeks before the swarm issues, because for a swarm to occur, colonies must produce one or more new queens. Ten days before swarming, workers engorge on honey to ensure they have sufficient energy reserves while in transit and while establishing their new nests.[67] Preceding swarming, workers also decrease their rate of dorsoventral vibrations, run back and forth across the comb in waves, and buzz to excite other workers,[68] with specific vibrational spectra being shown as predictive of when swarming will occur.[69] Workers will also chase, bite, and pull the queen along, eventually resulting in a mass of workers and the queen issuing from the colony. Normally younger workers, less than 10 days old, issue with swarms, leaving older workers and emerging brood in the original colony.[70] The first swarm of the season, known as the primary swarm, is composed of the old queen and approximately half the workers that leave the parental colony to establish a new one, leaving behind a series of virgin daughter queens and the remaining workers. The swarming bees will quickly exit the hive as a cloud until they amalgamate in a beardlike cluster at a temporary site, such as a tree branch or fencepost, where they collectively decide on their future nest site[66] (**Fig. 7**). The latter is accomplished through the action of scout bees who recruit nestmates using competing dances on the surface of the swarm itself[1]; once the swarm colonizes a site, the scouts release Nasonov pheromone as an attraction cue at the nest entrance.[66] After the primary swarms issue, the new virgins emerge about a week later, and once mated, the colony may produce one or two afterswarms or kill all but one remaining queen, which will mate and rule over the nest.[1] Considerable interaction exists between virgin queens and workers after the first queen emerges from her cell, primarily to prevent the emergence of more than one virgin at a time and to regulate fights between queens once swarming is completed.[71] The presence of a virgin in a colony suppresses the emergence of others by stimulating DVAV signals by workers on other mature queen cells, and by the emerged queen signaling her presence by pheromones and "piping".[1] Piping is a pulsed, high-pitched sound emitted by a queen causing workers to freeze in place and preventing them from chewing away wax and fibers on the ends of queen cells, thus delaying or preventing queen emergence. The piping signals produced by newly emerged queens are often referred to as *toots*. These signals are responded to by queens still confined in their cells by other piping signals called *quacks*, which are thought to alert the emerged queen to their presence. If two or more virgin queens are released at the same time, they may tolerate each other for several hours, but will inevitably fight to the death. When afterswarming is complete, emerged queens will kill queens still held within their cells.

A second type of reproduction in honey bee colonies is known as supersedure, in which the old queen is dispatched and, typically, no swarm is produced. Causes of supersedure include diminished pheromone production by the queen or the production of few or unfertilized eggs.[72] Consequently, older queens are more commonly

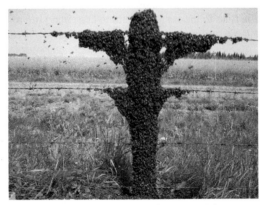

Fig. 7. A swarm temporarily alighting on a fencepost soon after issuing from the original nest.

superseded than younger queens. When supersedure occurs, colonies typically rear less than six queen cells and old the queen is often not eliminated until the successful virgin has begun her own egg laying.[1]

SUMMARY

Honey bee societies are highly evolved and have three distinct castes, with one reproductive queen normally present per colony. The queen lays all the eggs to produce new members and is at the apex of the social order for the hive. Workers in the colony are highly cooperative and progress through a series of within-hive tasks relating to brood and queen care, food storage and then later transition to outdoor tasks such as guarding and foraging. Honey bees have evolved a remarkable form of communication known as *dance language*, used to recruit other foragers to the location of food sources, yet also have the ability to communicate through the production of pheromones that regulate the efficiency and social order of the colony and maintain the queen's dominance. Colonies reproduce and disperse by swarming, at which time queens mate with multiple drones as a strategy to maximize overall colony fitness, productivity, and resilience to disease.

CLINICS CARE POINTS

- Veterinarians should endeavor to have a thorough understanding of honey bee biology to engage with beekeeping clients and distinguish between healthy and abnormal colonies.

- As queens age, their reproductive fitness decreases and their output of queen-produced pheromones diminishes. Regular replacement of queens (every 1–2 years) is a strategy to ensure high colony productivity and to avoid supersedure from occurring.

- Beekeepers actively manage against natural tendencies of colonies to swarm, so as to avoid disruptions in the colony life cycle leading to lowered productivity (ie, honey production), and to avoid losing bees to unknown locations.

DISCLOSURE

The author has nothing to disclose.

REFERENCES

1. Winston ML. The biology of the honey bee. Cambridge (MA): Harvard University Press; 1987.
2. Caron DM. Honey bee biology and beekeeping. Cheshire (CT): Wicwas Press; 1999.
3. Tarpy DR, Nielsen R, Nielsen DI. A scientific note on the revised estimates of effective paternity frequency in Apis. Insectes Soc 2004;51:203–4.
4. Withrow JM, Tarpy DR. Cryptic "royal" subfamilies in honey bee (*Apis mellifera*) colonies. PLoS One 2018;13(7):e0199124.
5. Mattila HR, Seeley TD. Genetic diversity in honey bee colonies enhances productivity and fitness. Science 2007;317:362–4.
6. Seeley TD, Tarpy DR. Queen promiscuity lowers disease within honeybee colonies. Proc Biol Sci 2007;274:67–72.
7. Seeley TD. Honeybee ecology: a study of adaptation in social life. Princeton (NJ): Princeton University Press; 1985.

8. Ribbands CR. The behaviour and social life of honeybees. London: Bee Research Association Ltd.; 1953.

9. Fukuda H, Sekiguchi K. Seasonal change of the honeybee worker longevity in Sapporo, North Japan, with notes on some factors affecting the life-span. Jap J Ecol 1966;16:206–12.

10. Anderson J. Proceedings of the conference. How long does a bee live? Bee World 1931;12:25–6.

11. Farrar CL. Arena. Bee World 1949;30:51.

12. Koeniger G, Koeniger N, Fabritius M. Some detailed observations of mating in the honeybee. Bee World 1979;60:53–7.

13. Baudry E, Solignac M, Garnery L, et al. Relatedness among honeybees (Apis mellifera) of a drone congregation. Proc Roy Soc B 1998;265(1409):2009–14.

14. Koeniger G. Mating sign and multiple mating in the honeybee. Bee World 1986; 67:141–50.

15. Michner CD. The social behavior of the bees. Cambridge (MA): Belknap Press of Harvard University Press; 1974.

16. Wilson EO. The insect societies. Cambridge (MA): Belknap Press of Harvard University Press; 1971.

17. Wilson EO. Sociobiology: the new synthesis. Cambridge (MA): Belknap Press of Harvard University Press; 1975.

18. Meunier J. Social immunity and the evolution of group living in insects. Phil Trans R Soc Lond B Biol Sci 2015;370(1669):20140102.

19. Bonoan RE, Iglesias Feliciano PM, Chang J, et al. Social benefits require a community: the influence of colony size on behavioral immunity in honey bees. Apidologie 2020;51:701–9.

20. von Frisch K. The dance language and orientation of bees. Cambridge (MA): Harvard University Press; 1967.

21. Dyer FC, Gould JL. Honey bee navigation. Am Sci 1983;71:587–97.

22. Dyer FC. The biology of the dance language. Annu Rev Entomol 2002;47:917–49.

23. Riley JR, Greggers U, Smith AD, et al. The flight paths of honeybees recruited by the waggle dance. Nature 2005;435:205–7.

24. Hopkins CY, Jevans AW, Boch R. Occurrence of octadeca-trans-2,cis-9,cis-12-trienoic acid in pollen attractive to the honey bee. Can J Biochem 1969;47:433–6.

25. Seeley TD. The wisdom of the hive: the social physiology of honey bee colonies. Harvard (MA): Harvard University Press; 1995.

26. Nieh JC. The honey bee shaking signal: function and design of a modulatory communication signal. Behav Ecol Sociobiol 1998;42:23–36.

27. Schneider SS, Lewis LA. The vibration signal, modulatory communication and the organization of labor in honey bees, Apis mellifera. Apidologie 2004;35:117–31.

28. Ramsey M, Bencsik M, Newton MI. Extensive vibrational characterisation and long-term monitoring of honeybee dorso-ventral abdominal vibration signals. Sci Rep 2018;8:14571.

29. Free JB. Pheromones of social bees. London: Chapman and Hall; 1987.

30. Nation JL. Insect physiology and biochemistry. Boca Raton (FL): CRC Press, Inc.; 2002.

31. Slessor KN, Kaminski LA, King GGS, et al. Semiochemical basis of the retinue response to queen honey bees. Nature 1988;332:354–6.

32. Kaminski LA, Slessor KN, Winston ML, et al. Honeybee response to queen mandibular pheromone in laboratory bioassays. J Chem Ecol 1990;16:841–50.

33. Slessor KN, Winston ML, Le Conte Y. Pheromone communication in the honeybee (Apis mellifera L.). J Chem Ecol 2005;31:2731–45.

34. Keeling CI, Slessor KN, Higo HA, et al. New components of the honey bee (*Apis mellifera* L.) queen retinue pheromone. Proc Natl Acad Sci U S A 2003;100: 4486–91.

35. Hoover SE, Keeling CI, Winston ML, et al. The effect of queen pheromones on worker honey bee ovary development. Naturwissenschaften 2003;90:477–80.

36. Higo HA, Winston ML, Slessor KN. Mechanisms by which honey bee (Hymenoptera: Apidae) queen pheromone sprays enhance pollination. Ann Entomol Soc Am 1992;88:366–73.

37. Ledoux M, Winston M, Higo H, et al. Queen and pheromonal factors influencing comb construction by simulated honey bee (*Apis mellifera* L.) swarms. Insectes Soc 2001;48:14–20.

38. Bortolotti L, Costa C. Chemical communication in the honey bee society. In: Mucignat-Caretta C, editor. Neurobiology of chemical communication. Boca Raton (FL): CRC Press/Taylor & Francis; 2014. p. 147–210.

39. Jay SC. Factors influencing ovary development of worker honeybees under natural conditions. Can J Zool 1968;46:345–7.

40. Mohammedi A, Paris A, Crauser D, et al. Effect of aliphatic esters on ovary development of queenless bees (*Apis mellifera* L.). Naturwissenschaften 1998;85: 455–8.

41. Naumann K, Winston ML, Slessor KN, et al. Production and transmission of honey bee queen (*Apis mellifera* L.) mandibular gland pheromone. Behav Ecol Sociobiol 1991;29:321–32.

42. Naumann K, Winston ML, Slessor KN. Movement of honey bee (*Apis mellifera* L.) queen mandibular gland pheromone in populous and unpopulous colonies. J Insect Behav 1993;6:211–23.

43. Winston ML, Slessor KN, Willis LG, et al. The influence of queen mandibular pheromones on worker attraction to swarm clusters and inhibition of queen rearing in the honey bee (*Apis mellifera* L.). Insectes Soc 1989;36:15–27.

44. Pickett JA, Williams IH, Martin AP. (Z)-11-eicosen-1-ol, an important new pheromonal component from the sting of the honey bee, *Apis mellifera* L. (Hymenoptera, Apidae). J Chem Ecol 1982;8:163–75.

45. Free JB, Williams IH. Exposure of the Nasonov gland by honeybees (*Apis mellifera*) collecting water. Behaviour 1970;37:286–90.

46. Free JB, Williams IH. The role of the Nasonov gland pheromone in crop communication by honeybees (*Apis mellifera* L.). Behaviour 1972;41:314–8.

47. Al-Kahtani SN, Bienefeld K. The Nasonov gland pheromone is involved in recruiting honey bee workers for individual larvae to be reared as queens. J Insect Behav 2012;25:392–400.

48. Lensky Y, Cassier P, Finkel A, et al. The fine structure of the tarsal glands of the honey bee *Apis mellifera* L. (Hymenoptera). Cell Tissue Res 1985;240:153–8.

49. Williams IH, Pickett JA, Martin AP. The Nasonov pheromone of the honeybee *Apis mellifera* L. (Hymenoptera, Apidae). Part II. Bioassay of the components using foragers. J Chem Ecol 1981;7:225–37.

50. Ferguson AW, Free JB. Factors determining the release of Nasonov pheromone by honey bees at the hive entrance. Physiol Entomol 1981;6:15–9.

51. Blum MS, Fales HM, Tucker KW, et al. Chemistry of the sting apparatus of the worker honey bee. J Apic Res 1978;17:218–21.

52. Boch R, Shearer DA, Stone BC. Identification of iso-amyl acetate as an active component in the sting pheromone of the honey bees. Nature 1962;195:1018–20.

53. Shearer DA, Boch R. 2-Heptanone in the mandibular gland secretion of the honey bee. Nature 1965;206:530.

54. Balderrama N, Nuñez J, Guerrieri F, et al. Different functions of two alarm substances in the honey bee. J Comp Physiol A 2002;188:485–91.
55. Collins AM, Rinderer T, Daly HV, et al. Alarm pheromone production by two honey bee (*Apis mellifera*) types. J Chem Ecol 1989;15:1747–56.
56. Hunt GJ, Wood KV, Guzmán-Novoa E, et al. Discovery of 3-methyl-2-buten-1-yl acetate, a new alarm component in the sting apparatus of Africanized honey bees. J Chem Ecol 2003;29:451–61.
57. Le Conte Y, Arnold G, Trouiller J, et al. Identification of a brood pheromone in honey bees. Naturwissenschaften 1990;77:334–6.
58. Le Conte Y, Sreng L, Trouiller J. The recognition of larvae by worker honey bees. Naturwissenschaften 1994;81:462–5.
59. Mohammedi A, Crauser D, Paris A, et al. Effect of a brood pheromone on honey bee hypopharyngeal glands. C R Acad Sci III 1996;319:769–72.
60. Le Conte Y, Sreng L, Poitout SH. Brood pheromone can modulate the feeding behavior of *Apis mellifera* workers (Hymenoptera: Apidae). J Econ Entomol 1995;88:798–804.
61. Pankiw T, Roman R, Sagili RR, et al. Brood pheromone effects on colony protein supplement consumption and growth in the honey bee (Hymenoptera: Apidae) in a subtropical winter climate. J Econ Entomol 2008;101:1749–55.
62. Pankiw T, Roman R, Sagili RR, et al. Pheromone-modulated behavioral suites influence colony growth in the honey bee (*Apis mellifera*). Naturwissenschaften 2004;91:575–8.
63. Sagili RR, Pankiw T. Effects of brood pheromone modulated brood rearing behaviors on honey bee (*Apis mellifera* L.) colony growth. J Insect Behav 2009;22:339–49.
64. Maisonnasse A, Lenoir JC, Beslay D, et al. E-β-ocimene, a volatile brood pheromone involved in social regulation in the honey bee colony (*Apis mellifera*). PLoS One 2010b;5(10):e13531.
65. Le Conte Y, Mohammedi A, Robinson GE. Primer effects of a brood pheromone on honey bee behavioural development. Proc R Soc Lond B 2001;268:163–8.
66. Seeley TD, Buhrman SC. Group decision making in swarms of honey bees. Behav Ecol Sociobiol 1999;45:19–31.
67. Combs GF. The engorgement of swarming worker honeybees. J Apic Res 1971;11:121–8.
68. Fletcher DJC. Significance of dorsoventral abdominal vibration among honeybees (*Apis mellifera* L.). Nature 1975;256:721–3.
69. Ramsey M-T, Bencsik M, Newton MI, et al. The prediction of swarming in honeybee colonies using vibrational spectra. Sci Rep 2020;10:9798.
70. Winston ML, Otis GW. Ages of bees in swarms and afterswarms of the Africanized honeybee. J Apic Res 1978;17:123–9.
71. Grooters HJ. Influences of queen piping and worker behaviour on the timing of emergence of honeybee queens. Insectes Soc 1987;34:181–93.
72. Butler CD. The process of queen supersedure in colonies of honeybees (*Apis mellifera* Linn.). Insectes Soc 1957;4:211–23.

Diseases and Pests of Honey Bees (*Apis Mellifera*)

Deborah J.M. Pasho, DVM[a,b,]*, Jeffrey R. Applegate Jr, DVM, DACZM[c,d,e], Don I. Hopkins[f,g]

KEYWORDS

- Foulbrood • Varroa • Fungal • Nosema • Deformed wing virus • Small hive beetle
- Wax moth

KEY POINTS

- American foulbrood is an infectious bacterial disease in honey bees caused by *Paenibacillus larvae*, which primarily affects capped brood through highly contagious spores.
- European foulbrood is caused by the nonsporulating bacterium *Melissococcus plutonius*, which generally affects open brood at times of increased hive stress and poor nutrition.
- *Varroa destructor* is a pervasive external parasite of honey bees that not only causes significant injury through feeding on the bees' fat bodies but also weakens and destroys colonies through vectoring of several viruses.
- Fungal diseases, namely Stonebrood and Chalkbrood, can destroy a colony, yet most often they can be resolved through increased ventilation, nutrition, and interhive hygiene without significant colony loss.
- Five of the six viral infections reviewed here are vectored by *Varroa destructor* and together cause parasitic mite syndrome to include weakening of the colony, bee death, and significant colony losses.
- Nosema is a microsporidial disease that is associated with diarrhea and can often be managed with good nutrition.

BACTERIAL
American Foulbrood

American foulbrood (AFB) is a contagious and infectious disease of honey bees that affects the capped brood. It is caused by the bacteria, *Paenibacillus larvae*, which

[a] Huckleberry Farm Bee Services, P.O. Box 173, Hartland, VT 05048, USA; [b] Honey Bee Veterinary Consortium, 3912 Battleground Avenue, Suite 112 PMB# 154, Greensboro, NC 27410, USA; [c] Nautilus Avian and Exotics Veterinary Specialists, 1010 Falkenberg Road, Brick, NJ 08724, USA; [d] Honey Bee Veterinary Consortium, 3912 Battleground Avenue, Suite 112 PMB# 154, Greensboro, NC 27410, USA; [e] Department of Clinical Sciences, North Carolina State University, College of Veterinary Medicine, 1060 William Moore Drive Raleigh, NC 27607, USA; [f] 381 Griffin Rd, Snow Camp, NC 27349, USA; [g] North Carolina Department of Agriculture and Consumer Services, Plant Industry Division, 1001 Mail Service Center, Raleigh, NC 27699-1001, USA
* Corresponding author. Huckleberry Farm Bee Services, P.O. Box 173, Hartland, VT 05048.
E-mail address: dpasho@hotmail.com

Vet Clin Food Anim 37 (2021) 401–412
https://doi.org/10.1016/j.cvfa.2021.06.001
0749-0720/21/© 2021 Elsevier Inc. All rights reserved.

vetfood.theclinics.com

has both vegetative and spore forms. Spores are the infectious form and reportedly remain viable for more than 10 years in the environment and on equipment, withstanding extreme environmental conditions.[1] The Beltsville bee laboratory installed combs that had been set aside for more than 70 years; the resulting colony breakdown demonstrated that the spores were still viable.[2] This serious disease is reportable in many countries and has the potential to result in devastating losses. The bacteria are introduced into the colony when adults become infected with spores, commonly via contaminated equipment and tools. Spores, unknowingly mixed in with brood food, are fed to larvae.[1] The infectious dose is as little as 10 spores in a 12- to 36-hour-old larva.[3] Once ingested, the spores are activated into their vegetative form, which kills the larva, metabolizing it into the characteristic viscous, brown material. Once the vegetative form of the bacteria has exhausted its nutrient supply, spores are formed creating the dried-up, dark brown, hard-to-remove scale.[1] If AFB is not caught, the queen will lay more eggs in the "empty," spore-laden brood cells, and the new larvae will be infected by millions of bacterial spores already present in their brood cells. Another wave of brood will fail to mature; the hive will quickly become fully infected, resulting in a potential AFB nidus for the apiary.

Clinical signs consist of a distinctive foul odor, a spotty "shotgun" brood pattern, sunken (**Fig. 1**) and greasy-looking brood cell caps, cappings that are perforated (from nurse bees opening the cells after detecting infection), caramel-colored and viscous larvae having a ropiness that can be drawn out with a matchstick, dried hard dark scale in the brood cell, and rarely a dried-up pupa with its proboscis (tongue) sticking to the opposite wall.[4] The well-adhered hard scale is found at the lower edges of cells and can be seen by holding the frame horizontally with the top bar toward the holder. Interestingly, the scales will fluoresce under black light.[5]

There are several diseases with similar appearance that should be included on the differential diagnosis list. European foulbrood, another bacterial disease, can affect capped brood during severe infection yet has a distinctly different malodor than AFB. Parasitic mite syndrome and idiopathic brood disease are not bacterial, although they can also present with spotty brood patterns.

A colony with apparent field symptoms of AFB should not be treated with antibiotics. The colony should be depopulated and the equipment disposed of in a manner that will ensure no other bees are exposed to this source of infection. Treating the

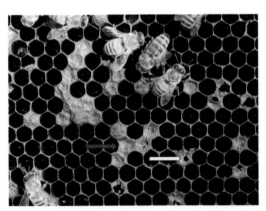

Fig. 1. American foulbrood clinical signs: "shotgun" brood pattern, perforated caps (*white arrow*), sunken caps (*red arrow*), and lack of diseased open brood. (*Courtesy of* Don Hopkins, Raleigh NC.)

remaining colonies in the apiaries with a one-time prophylactic antimicrobial treatment may be considered. Close follow-up is required. There are currently 3 antimicrobials labeled by Food and Drug Administration (FDA) to address the issue of AFB. They are oxytetracycline (Terramycin), tylosin, and lincomycin. Tylosin and lincomycin were approved for cases where the bacteria were expressing resistance to oxytetracycline. All 3 antibiotics are intended to inhibit the expression of the vegetative stage; any *P larvae* spores remaining will not be affected.

European Foulbrood

European foulbrood (EFB) is caused by the gram-positive bacterium *Melissococcus plutonius*. It often shows up late spring to early summer[4] when colonies are deficient in protein and there are not enough nurse bees to provide for the larvae.[6] Other associated stressors that predispose to EFB infection are confinement secondary to poor weather or prolonged transport and concurrent infections with sacbrood bee virus and *Varroa destructor*.[1] Unlike *P larvae*, *M plutonius* does not produce spores and mostly affects uncapped, not capped, brood. Larvae usually succumb to the bacterial infection at 4 to 5 days of age[7] after consuming bacteria-laden food.[4] It should be noted, occasionally larvae die after capping, and sunken caps can be seen, leading to the differential diagnosis of AFB.[8]

Clinical signs of EFB include a low population, spotty brood pattern, larval discoloration (progressing from yellow to gray),[7] and a visible tracheal tube[4] (**Fig. 2**). European foulbrood is usually not present in a colony infected with AFB due to production of an antibiotic produced by the *P larvae* that prevents coinfection.[8] Infected larvae are seen in a twisted position rather than the standard C shape at the bottom of the cells.[4] There can be a malodor present and dry, rubbery, easily removed scales can be seen inside the cells.

Because EFB is not as contagious as AFB, it is not necessary to remove the colony from the apiary immediately. There are steps that can be taken to remedy the situation and allow the colony to return to a healthy, strong, and productive colony of bees. If caught early enough, simple steps such as feeding a supplemental diet or moving the hive to a better food source may be enough. It is known that *Melissococcus plutonis* competes for the nutrition that the bee is fed in its developmental stages, and the larva is essentially starved. Thus, by providing supplemental food or nectar sources, the bees may be able to overcome the infection on their own. Requeening or breaking

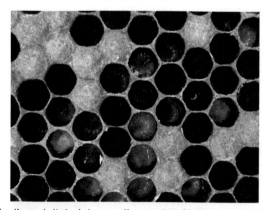

Fig. 2. European foulbrood clinical signs: yellow, twisted larvae, some with a visible tracheal tube. (*Courtesy of* Amy Franklin.)

the brood cycle is another simple step that may help the bees overcome EFB. With no more eggs being laid by a queen, and thus no more infected larvae being produced, the workers have more time to clean up and drag out the infected larvae. Because there is less of a pool of infection in the colony, when the queen resumes egg laying, the workers will be able to rear healthy larvae; this is also true with replacing the queen, and in addition, the new queen may have genetics that are more tolerable of this disease.

In the case of AFB, the common state/provincial regulations are not to treat but to depopulate the colony. With EFB there are treatment options: breaking the brood cycle, requeening, moving the colony, or feeding a supplemental diet. The use of antibiotics should be a last resort. The only antibiotic available for this purpose is oxytetracycline. The standard regime would be to dust along the edge of the top bars with a 200 mg dose followed weekly for 2 more weeks for a total of 600 mg per hive. See label for more precise instructions.

PARASITES AND PESTS
Varroosis

Varroa destructor is an external parasite of honey bees. It is visible with the naked eye as an oval, red-brown colored, flat disc with 8 legs (**Fig. 3**). Female *Varroa* enter a cell just before capping and lays one male egg and subsequent female eggs. They hatch, molt several times, and then breed together within the still-sealed cell.[1] Women exit the cell when the adult bee ecloses (emerges from the brood cell). *Varroa* are spread between colonies, whereas in their phoretic phase on adult bees, through robbing of and drifting to nearby hives. *Varroa destructor* feeds off the fat bodies[9] of developing and adult bees with its reproductive life cycle taking place exclusively in capped cells.[10] Not only does the direct feeding of the varroa mite weaken all stages of bee development but also viruses such as deformed wing virus (DWV), acute bee paralysis virus, Kashmir bee virus, Israeli acute paralysis virus, and slow bee paralysis virus are vectored by *Varroa*.[11]

The pathogenesis causes decreased weight in adult bees,[11] decreased lifespan,[12] shortened abdomen, crippled wings (due to transmission of DWV),[11] impaired navigational abilities,[13] immunosuppression, and decreased drone reproduction ability.[1]

Clinical signs can be characterized by the term parasitic mite syndrome, which is the compilation of clinical signs from the combination of *Varroa* infestation and DWV. These signs consist of decreased population and honey production,[1] deformed wings due to the associated DWV, winter death of the colony despite adequate food stores

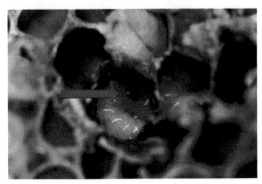

Fig. 3. *Varroa destructor* seen on a larva. (*Courtesy of* Don Hopkins, Raleigh NC.)

and ventilation, and visible mites on adult bees. In addition, grainy mite feces, or white guanine deposits, can be seen with high infestation on the top side of the cells and are visible if the frame is held horizontally with the top bar farther away from the holder.[7] A large colony can handle this type of loss in small numbers, but as the mite population increases, the larger number of deaths begins to take a toll and the population of honey bees begins to decline. Treatment should address the varroa mite issue with a regime using one of the approved miticides following label directions. The efficacy of the treatment will depend on the level of infestation.

Wax Moths

The greater wax moth (*Galleria mellonella*) is an insect that tends to only affect colonies weakened by a primary stressor and can be especially problematic in stored equipment. They breed outside of the hive and then female wax moths lay eggs inside the hive in crevices where bees cannot reach them for removal.[7] Up to 600 eggs can be laid at one time.[14] Once hatched, larvae move through the hive, in a protective tunnel of their own web, destroying the comb. The larvae eat and/or damage wax, honey, pollen, larval skins, and wooden ware while producing hive detritus.[15,16] Interestingly, *G mellonella* has been found to be able to consume, degrade, and derive energy from low-density polyethylene,[17] which could be beneficial for plastic decomposition.

Clinical signs consist of observing white to gray larva ranging in size from 1 to 20 mm long that tunnel through wax comb and make webs within the wax[18] (**Fig. 4**). The honey bee brood may also be eaten by the voracious *G mellonella* larva. Differential diagnosis is small hive beetle (SHB) larvae, yet no web will be seen with SHB larvae.

The lesser wax moth (*Achroia grisella*) is less prevalent and smaller than the greater wax moth. Its larvae cause damage to bee larvae differently than *G mellonella* and is evident by straight burrowed galleries just below the brood cell cappings. Nurse bees then uncap the damaged bee larvae, and the exposed larvae is known as "bald brood." *Achroia grisella* is controlled the same way as *G mellonella*.[1]

Small Hive Beetle

Small hive beetles (*Athena tumida*) are notorious pests that destroy wax comb, honey, and pollen stores when feeding during the larval stage. These beetles are an introduced pest from southern Africa, first identified in the United States in Florida in

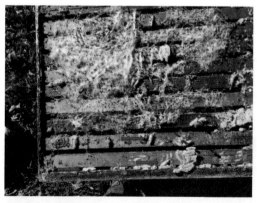

Fig. 4. Wax moth infestation. Notice white webbing and larvae (*arrows*). (*Courtesy of* Don Hopkins, Raleigh NC.)

1998. Subsequent investigation shows a previous discovery 2 years earlier in South Carolina, most likely arriving by ship at Savanna or Charleston, that was not identified at that time.[19] The preferred diet of the beetle is found inside the honey bee colony, but they can survive on other food sources, such as fruits, because they belong to the sap beetle family (Nitidulidae).

Adult beetles enter the hive to lay eggs in inaccessible cracks, where bees can remove neither the eggs nor the adults. The bees confine and guard the beetles in these inaccessible "prisons," yet the beetles do not starve because they are continuously fed via bee-trophylaxis stimulated by stroking the bees' mandibles.[20] Up to 2000 eggs are laid by an SHB in its lifetime, and eggs develop in 3 to 6 days, depending on environmental conditions, creating an overwhelming amount of destruction.[21] The SHB larvae will then feed on all the resources within the colony, including the honey, pollen, and bee brood, causing quite a disruption to the bees. A strong honey bee colony is able to handle the pressure of the beetles; however, under the right conditions, a colony of honey bees will succumb to the beetles within a few days. After about 7 days of feeding, the larvae then leave the hive and wander to find suitable soil in which to pupate.[22] Pupation can take 21 days, at which point the adults emerge from the soil and search for a new hive to invade.

Clinical signs consist of damaged frames from not only the mechanical larval eating, but also from an orange-smelling slime produced from a combination of fermenting honey and SHB larval defecation. The adult beetles and larvae will be observed in the hive, and the bees may abscond an infested hive[8] (**Fig. 5**). Differential diagnosis is *G mellonella*, the greater wax moth, and the lesser wax moth (*A grisella*).

There are several devices available to control small hive beetles; however, none seem to be terribly effective. Some may help keep the population numbers reduced but will not eradicate this pest. The 2 things most helpful in preventing beetle problems are placement of the hive in direct sunlight and limiting the empty space in the hive. There should not be more space than the bees can protect, so the hive size should equal the nest size to limit beetles' free space.

Most beekeepers do not consider the beetle to be a major threat to their apiary. However, anything that affects the colony dynamics can cause a cascading event leading to the disruption of the colony. There is evidence that the beetle, such as the varroa mite, might be a vector of some of the bacterial and viral pathogens affecting the bees. More research on the direct and indirect impact of the SHB is needed.

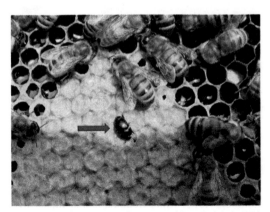

Fig. 5. Adult small hive beetle. (*Courtesy of* Don Hopkins, Raleigh NC.).

Tracheal Mites

Tracheal mites (*Acarapis woodi*) are a parasite of the trachea of the 3 adult honey bee castes, with a preference for drones.[23] Tracheal mites infest adult honey bees that are 10 to 15 day old by entering through the spiracles and gaining access to the tracheal network.[23] Individual affected bees may be unable to fly and can be found crawling on the ground or dead near the hive entrance. At the hive level, seen mainly in the spring, there are decreases in population, brood, and honey stores.[23] Diagnosis is made by removing the head and first set of legs, obliquely cutting off a small segment of the thorax containing the tracheal tube, and visualizing mites under the microscope. There has been a decline in the number of tracheal mites detected at the USDA-ARS bee laboratory in Beltsville, MD,[24] which may have to do with the coinciding effective treatment of *Varroa*.

FUNGAL
Chalkbrood

Chalkbrood disease, caused by the opportunistic fungus *Ascosphaera apis*, affects colonies seasonally in the cool spring when weather is damp and while populations of brood are increasing, although it can occur at other times in the year. Low numbers of nurse bees from overwintering and insufficient brood warmth are stressors to a rebuilding spring colony. During this and other times of hive stress, such as poor nutrition, in-hive moisture buildup, and weakness from other diseases, the brood are susceptible to infection. *A apis* can be transmitted to other colonies by use of contaminated equipment and tools, shared food sources, and robbing by other bees.

It is introduced to larva when spores are fed in contaminated bee bread to brood. These spores germinate in the intestines of the larva that triggers the formation of mycelium. The mycelium grows to invade adjacent tissue and eventually penetrates all tissues of the larvae. Infected, yet asymptomatic, larvae are capped, and death occurs within the first 2 days of the pupal stage.[25]

Clinical signs include a weakened colony that has a decreased population. The pupae become mummified and covered in white, gray, or black mycelium resembling a piece of chalk when white (**Fig. 6**). The mummified pupae are often found on the bottom board or at the entrance of the hive due to removal by housekeeping workers. Capped cells may be perforated, and moldy dead pupae can be seen in the cells.[1]

Diagnosis is by observation of mold in brood cells and the presence of mummified pupa in the hive. Research by Khan and colleagues (2020) showed that decreased levels of aerobic gut bacteria predict chalkbrood development, whereas increased levels of gut bacteria signal a recovery from the infection. Also suggested in the same study was potential for development of a probiotic treatment.[26]

There are no chemical treatments registered for use, and chalkbrood will usually clear up on its own. Adjustments that could be attempted include moving the hive to a warmer, drier environment, supplemental feeding, and adding healthy brood. Symptoms can clear up as quickly as the length of a brood cycle, if proper steps are taken. Caging the queen to break the brood cycle may help, or even replacing the queen in hopes of improving genetics as a genetic factor related to chalkbrood has been demonstrated.

Stonebrood

Stonebrood disease, caused by fungi of the genus *Aspergillus*, can infect all stages of bee development. Infections occur when spores are ingested through normal feeding practices and via fungal penetration of the cuticle.[27] This saprophytic fungus usually resides in soil and can also be pathogenic for birds and mammals, including humans, via carcinogenic aflatoxins, making beekeeper precaution and awareness essential.

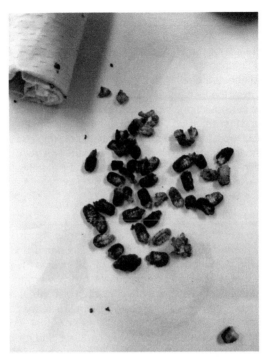

Fig. 6. Chalkbrood: shriveled, black/gray/white larvae. (*Courtesy of* Deborah Pasho, DVM.)

Tests show that the fungus is pervasive and highly infectious in the apiary, yet the prevalence of disease is rare and not well understood.[28]

Clinical signs include larvae covered in fluffy white mold that may turn yellow or greenish brown depending on the *Aspergillus* species. The larvae ultimately become hardened, stonelike, and difficult to crush. Adult bee symptoms are weakness, agitation, paralysis, and abdominal distension followed by death and subsequent mummification. Infection can cause death of the entire colony, but usually the disease spontaneously resolves. Stonebrood can be avoided if hives are kept dry and good husbandry practices are used: no shared equipment, use of clean tools, retiring old combs, etc.[29] Diagnosis is through laboratory analysis.

VIRAL
Acute Bee Paralysis Virus, Chronic Bee Paralysis Virus, Israeli Acute Paralysis Virus, Slow Bee Paralysis Virus

Acute bee paralysis virus (ABPV), chronic bee paralysis virus (CBPV), Israeli acute paralysis virus (IAPV), and slow bee paralysis virus are all RNA viruses that cause various forms of paralysis in bees through natural and experimental infections. All viruses are associated with *Varroa,* which acts as a vector, except for CBPV, which is transmitted through contact of feces in wounds.[1] In addition to paralysis and subsequent death, clinical signs include trembling, cessation of flight, black hairless abdomens (CBPV and IAPV) and rapid death (ABPV).[30] Diagnosis relies on clinical signs and laboratory testing but may be cost prohibitive for the beekeeper. Management and treatment are similar as with other viruses, by decreasing *Varroa* infestation,[31] good hygienic practices with equipment and tools, and providing good nutrition to increase hive health.

Deformed Wing Virus

Deformed wing virus (DWV) is a contagious virus belonging to family of Iflaviridae that causes widespread occurrence of shriveled deformed wings in the capped pupae before they emerge from cells as adults. The flightless adult also presents cognitive disabilities[32] and rounded shortened abdomens.[1] Although *Varroa destructor* is recently thought not to be responsible for viral replication,[33] it is recognized as a substantial mechanical vector for the transmission of the virus within the hive and to other hives.[34] Deformed wings indicate massive infestation by *Varroa*[35] and accompany other associated signs of parasitic mite syndrome.[36] Treatment consists of controlling and reducing *Varroa* mite infestation.

Sacbrood

Sacbrood virus belongs to the Iflaviridae family, along with DWV, slow brood paralysis virus, Kakugo virus, and Varroa destructor virus-1.[37] Larvae become infected when adults feed them with clinically normal, yet infected, hypopharyngeal glands, which in-turn infects other nurse bees as they detect, uncap, and remove infected deceased larvae. *Varroa destructor* and pollen are also thought to be vectors and fomites of the virus, respectively.[38] Although the latent infection in adults possibly only presents as decreased longevity,[39] infected larvae are yellow, stretched, uncapped, and seem as fluid-filled sacs[1] due to ecdysial fluid collecting beneath a failed pupation's unshed skin (**Fig. 7**). This later becomes a brown scale.[40] Differential diagnosis should include AFB, EFB, and brood mycosis.[1] Although there is no specific treatment of sacbrood, management includes increasing colony-health by using good equipment hygiene and providing good nutrition. Requeening with a more hygienic queen may also help.

MICROSPORIDIAL
Nosema

Nosemosis is an infection of the honey bee's digestive system caused by the Microsporidiae, *Nosema apis* (type A nosemosis) and *Nosema ceranae* (type C nosemosis), which are reported in 24 countries.[41] They are unicellular, obligate symbionts of animals, that used to be classified as protist, but were reclassified in 2005 as a reduced lineage of fungi,[42] and most recently in 2020 were placed into the new genus of Vairimorpha.[41,43]

On eating *Nosema* spores, the midgut becomes infected, spores are reproduced, and eventually the spores are collected in the lumen of the ventriculus and are evacuated in feces, thus enabling transmission to other bees.[1]

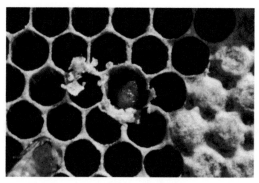

Fig. 7. Sacbrood virus clinical signs: stretched and discolored larva. (*Courtesy of* Don Hopkins, Raleigh NC.)

In general, clinical signs can be nonspecific or consist of diarrhea seen on combs, landing boards, and/or hive bodies. There can also be weakness, crawling bees, and death of worker bees.[5] Type C nosemosis tends to be asymptomatic and without a seasonal pattern.[5,44–46] Nosema type A infections affect already weakened colonies, leading to further damage of the colony. Predisposing influences include hive confinement, such as during times of prolonged inclement weather, overwintering, and commercial-related practices.[10]

Disease management consists of supplying good nutrition, using good inter-hive biosecurity, reducing environmental stressors, and performing careful inspections, thus limiting the spread secondarily from crushed bees. At the time of this writing, Fumigillin, with the trade name Fumidil-B, is reportedly effective against *N apis*, although not approved by the FDA.

CLINICS CARE POINTS

- AFB is a devastating disease to honey bees; due to the virulence and transmissibility of the disease and gravity of the subsequent management (destroying the colony and hive), it needs to be high on the rule out list.
- European foulbrood is considered less devastating that AFB and may be effectively managed multimodally with nutritional support, requeening for improved hygiene, and/or antimicrobial therapy.
- Varroosis is considered the most significant detriment to honey bee colonies. Varroa mites need to be controlled for successful colony survival.

DISCLOSURE

The authors have nothing to disclose.

REFERENCES

1. Vidal-Naquet N. Honeybee veterinary medicine: Apis mellifera L. Sheffield, United Kingdom: 5m Publishing; 2015.
2. Shimanuki H, Knox D. A. Diagnosis of honey bee diseases. Agriculture handbook, agricultural research service, 690. Beltsville, MD: US Department of Agriculture; 1991. p. 53.
3. Genersch E. American Foulbrood in honeybees and its causative agent, Paenibacillus larvae. J Invertebr Pathol 2010;103:S10–9.
4. Alippi A. Bee diseases (pathogenesis, epidemiology, diagnosis, therapy and prophylaxis). In: Ritter W, editor. Bee health and veterinarians. Paris: OIE; 2014. p. 117–24.
5. Lopez-Uribe M, Underwood R. Honey bee diseases: American Foulbrood. In: Penn state extension. 2019. Available at: https://extension.psu.edu/honey-bee-diseases-american-foulbrood. Accessed December 28, 2020.
6. Alippi A. Bacterial diseases. In: Colin ME, Ball BV, Kilani M, editors. Bee disease diagnosis. Options Mediterraneennes, Serie B. Etudes et Recherches, vol. 25. Zaragoza, Spain: CIHEAM Publications; 1999. Available at: http://om.ciheam.org/article.php?IDPDF=99600235.
7. Honey bees: a guide for veterinarians. Schaumburg, IL: American Veterinary Medical Association; 2017.

8. Caron D, Connor L. Honey bee biology and beekeeping. Pennsylvania: Wicwas Press, LLC; 2013. p. 341–9.

9. Ramsey S, Ochoa R, Bauchan G, et al. Varroa destructor feeds primarily on honey bee fat body tissue and not hemolymph. Proc Natl Acad Sci U S A 2020; 116(5):1792–801.

10. Applegate JRJr, Petritz OA. Common and emerging infectious diseases of honeybees (Apis mellifera). Vet Clin North Am Exot Anim Pract 2020;23(2):285–97.

11. Rosenkrantz P, Aumeier P, Ziegelmann B. Biology and control of Varroa destructor. J Invertebr Pathol 2010;103:96–119.

12. Schneider P, Drescher W. EInfluss der Parasitierung durch die Milbe Varroa jacobsoni aus das Schlupfgewicht, die Gewichtsentwicklung, die Entwicklung der Hypopharynxdrusen und die Lebensdauer von Apis mellifera. Apidologie 1987;18:101–6.

13. Kralj J, Brockmann A, Fuchs S, et al. The parasitic mite Varroa destructor affects non-associative learning in honey bee foragers, Apis mellifera L. J Comp Physiol A Neuroethol Sens Neural Behav Physiol 2007;193:363–70.

14. Ben Hamida B. Enemies of bees. In: Colin ME, Ball BV, Kilani M, editors. Bee disease diagnosis. Zaragoza: CIHEAM; 1999. p. 147–65. Available at: https://om.ciheam.org/om/pdf/b25/99600245.pdf (ciheam.org).

15. Mansour M. Radiation disinfestation of honeybee combs infested with greater wax moth eggs. J Apic Sci 2020;64(1):37–46.

16. Williams J. Insects: lepidoptera (moths). In: Honey bee pests, predators, and diseases, 3. Cambridge, Massachusetts: Harvard University Press; 1997. p. 119–42, 066-Williams–Insects; Lepidoptera (Moths).pdf (usda.gov).

17. LeMoine C, Grove H, Smith CM, et al. Very hungry caterpillar: polyethylene metabolism and lipid homeostasis in larvae of the greater wax moth (Galleria mellonella). Environ Sci Technol 2020;54(22):14706–15.

18. Kwadha CA, Ong'amo GO, Ndegwa PN, et al. The biology and control of the greater wax moth. Galleria Mellonella Insects 2017;8(2):61.

19. Hood W. Overview of the small hive beetle, Aethina tumida, in North America. Bee World 2000;81(3):129–37.

20. Shafer M, Ritter W. The small hive beetle. In: Ritter W, editor. Bee health and veterinarians. Paris: OIE; 2014. p. 149–56.

21. Akinwande K, Mogaji O, Alabi O. Survival and development of the small hive beetle, Aethina tumida, murray (coleoptera: nitidulidae), in the soil. Bee World 2020; 97(3):90–5.

22. Cuthbertson A, Wakefield M, Powell M, et al. The small hive beetle Aethina tumida: A review of its biology and control measures. Curr Zoolog 2013;59(5): 644–53.

23. Mondet F, Conte Y. Parasites. In: Ritter W, editor. Bee health and veterinarians. Paris: OIE; 2014. p. 131–41.

24. Moore P, Wilson M, Skinner J. Honey bee tracheal mites: gone? But not for good. Bee Health; 2019. Available at: https://bee-health.extension.org/Honey-Bee-Tracheal-Mites-Gone-But-not-for-Good. Accessed December 17, 2020.

25. Castagnino G, Jasna K, Brockmann A, et al. Etiology, symptoms and prevention of chalkbrood disease: a literature review. Rev Bras Saúde Prod Anim 2020;21: e210332020.

26. Khan S, Somerville D, Frese M, et al. Environmental gut bacteria in European honey bees (Apis mellifera) from Australia and their relationship to the chalkbrood disease. PLoS One 2020;15(8):e0238252.

27. Jensen A, Aronstein K, Flores J, et al. Standard methods for fungal brood disease research. J Apic Res 2013;52(1):1–20.

28. Foley K, Fazio G, Jensen A, et al. The distribution of Aspergillus spp. opportunistic parasites in hives and their pathogenicity to honey bees. Vet Microbiol 2014;169(3–4):203–10. Available at: http://www.sciencedirect.com/science/article/pii/S0378113513005531.

29. Chalkbrood and stonebrood. Food and agriculture organization of the United Nations. Source Apimondia, IZSLT - Istituto Zooprofilattico Sperimentale del Lazio e della Toscana "Mariano Aleandri". 2017. Available at: http://www.fao.org/3/ca4052en/ca4052en.pdf. Accessed December 19, 2020.

30. Dittes J, Aupperle-Lellbach H, Schäfer MO, et al. Veterinary diagnostic approach of common virus diseases in adult honeybees. Vet Sci 2020;7(4):159.

31. Dittes J, Schäfer MO, Aupperle-Lellbach H, et al. Overt infection with chronic bee paralysis virus (CBPV) in two honey bee colonies. Vet Sci 2020;7(3):142.

32. Javaid I, Uli M. Virus infection causes specific learning deficits in honeybee foragers. Proc R Soc B 2007;274:1517–21.

33. Brettell LE, Mordecai GJ, Schroeder DC, et al. A comparison of deformed wing virus in deformed and asymptomatic honey bees. Insects 2017;8(1):28.

34. Brettell L, Martin S. Oldest Varroa tolerant honey bee population provides insight into the origins of the global decline of honey bees. Sci Rep 2017;7:45953.

35. Ritter W. Viral diseases. In: Ritter W, editor. Bee health and veterinarians. Paris: World Organisation for Animal Health (OiE); 2014. p. 162.

36. Grozinger C, Underwood R, López-Uribe M. Viruses in honey bees. In: Penn state extension. 2020. Available at: https://extension.psu.edu/viruses-in-honey-bees. Accessed December 12, 2020.

37. Brutscher LM, McMenamin AJ, Flenniken ML. The buzz about honey bee viruses. PLoS Pathog 2016;12(8):e1005757.

38. Tantillo G, Bottaro M, Pinto A, et al. Virus infections of honeybees Apis mellifera. Ital J Food Saf 2015;4:157–68.

39. Yongsawas R, Chaimanee V, Pettis JS, et al. Impact of sacbrood virus on larval microbiome of Apis mellifera and Apis cerana. Insects 2020;11(7):439.

40. Grabensteiner E, Ritter W, Carter MJ, et al. Sacbrood virus of the honeybee (Apis mellifera): rapid identification and phylogenetic analysis using reverse transcription-PCR. Clin Diagn Lab Immunol 2001;8(1):93–104.

41. Grupe AC II, Quandt CA. A growing pandemic: a review of Nosema parasites in globally distributed domesticated and native bees. PLoS Pathog 2020;16(6): e1008580.

42. Adl S, Simpson A, Farmer M, et al. The new higher level classification of eukaryotes with emphasis on the taxonomy of protists. J Eukaryot Microbiol 2005;52: 399–451.

43. Tokarev YS, Huang WF, Solter LF, et al. A formal redefinition of the genera Nosema and Vairimorpha (Microsporidia: Nosematidae) and reassignment of species based on molecular phylogenetics. J Invertebr Pathol 2020;169:107279.

44. Fernandez JM, Puerta F, Cousinou M, et al. Asymptomatic presence of Nosema spp. in Spanish commercial apiaries. J Invertebr Pathol 2012;111:106–10.

45. Traver BE, Williams MR, Fell RD. Comparison of within hive sampling seasonal activity of Nosema ceranae in honey bee colonies. J Invertebr Pathol 2012;109: 187–93.

46. Fries I. Microsporidia. In: Ritter W, editor. Bee heath and veterinarians. Paris: OIE; 2014. p. 125–9.

Common Noninfectious Conditions of the Honey bees (*Apis mellifera*) Colony

Jeffrey R. Applegate Jr, DVM, DACZM[a,b,c,*]

KEYWORDS

- Starvation • Winter loss • Queenless laying worker hive • Hive microenvironment
- Overwintering • Chilled brood • Overheating • Humidity

KEY POINTS

- Starvation frequently is cited as a cause of colony loss, particularly over the winter.
- A queenless laying worker colony carries a poor prognosis and often results in a complete loss of the colony.
- Hive microclimate is complex, and minor intrahive changes of temperature and humidity can result in significant stress to the colony.

DISCUSSION

Starvation

Starvation is widely considered one of the leading causes of colony loss in overwintering hives, although it is not isolated to winter events and can occur in any season. There are 2 main reasons for winter starvation. First, bees perish due to inadequate honey stores going into the winter season, thus exhausting their rations prior to the spring nectar flow. Alternatively, the cluster simply gets separated from the honey supply within the hive, due to either physical separation or temperatures that remain too cold for the cluster to move to the stores.

National surveys are conducted to follow colony losses in the United States; between 2015 and 2016, total winter colony losses in the United States were reported as 26.9%, whereas summer colony loss was 23.6%.[1] At the time of this report, this was the third consecutive year that summer losses approximated winter losses,

[a] Nautilus Avian and Exotics Veterinary Specialists, 1010 Falkenberg Road, Brick, NJ 08724, USA; [b] Honey Bee Veterinary Consortium, Raleigh, North Carolina, USA; [c] Department of Clinical Sciences, North Carolina State University, College of Veterinary Medicine, Raleigh, North Carolina, USA
* Corresponding author. Nautilus Avian and Exotics Veterinary Specialists, 1010 Falkenberg Road, Brick, NJ 08724.
E-mail address: DrJeff@NAEVS.net

Vet Clin Food Anim 37 (2021) 413–425
https://doi.org/10.1016/j.cvfa.2021.06.002
0749-0720/21/© 2021 Elsevier Inc. All rights reserved.

although losses can vary annually. Colony losses for migratory beekeepers, ones who moved hives across state lines, trended lower than stationary beekeepers. Concurrently, hobbyist beekeepers experienced higher annual and winter losses than commercial beekeepers. Starvation was higher for backyard and sideline beekeepers than for commercial beekeepers for the reported 2015 to 2016 year as well as the 3 years prior.[1–4] Worldwide, losses vary widely, with Slovakia reporting winter losses as low as 10% annually between 2009 and 2015, ranking among countries lowest in winter mortality. Although starvation is expected as the leading cause, the reasons for the low number of losses are related to varroa mite management during summer, autumn, and winter periods combined with treatment during summer nectar flow with organic acids.[5]

Honey bee nutrition, in the form of honey stores, is a vital component of hive survival, particularly over winter. A worker bee requires 11 mg of dry sugar every day, which is equivalent to 22 microliter of 50% sugar syrup per worker per day. Maintenance for a strong summer hive of approximately 50,000 bees requires 1.1 L (approximately 2 lb) of 50% sugar per day,[6] although, due to decreased metabolism, less activity, and lower worker numbers, winter consumption needs are less. In a natural setting, if not managed on a floral monoculture, all the necessary nutrients can be acquired from native plants. Modern agriculture and monocropping may be harmful to the colony by not providing a varied and nutritionally complete diet, thus weakening a hive and potentially lowering the hive immunity causing increased susceptibility to threatening disease, such as European foulbrood and viral, fungal, and other diseases. With the exception of rapeseed, which appears to be an excellent singular food source, polyfloral pollen diets are superior to monocultures.

Environmental conditions can affect honey storage and nutrition. High ambient temperatures and sufficient precipitation are linked with increased foraging, whereas inclement weather confines workers to the hive.[7–11] Persistent unfavorable weather conditions can decrease foraging returns and stored honey resulting in a weakened hive.[7,12] Springtime starvation risks may be exacerbated by bad weather, including cold temperatures and spring rains (in temperate regions). The cold weather reduces foraging efforts due to the formation of an active cluster attempting to keep the larvae and queen warm, and the wet season may wash nectar from flowers, reducing the available forage for the bees. In summer, a nectar dearth results in less resources to forage as well, which can prove exceptionally challenging for a hive that recently has had honey harvested. The reduced foraging results in less food returned to the hive and, therefore, of a lack of resources (protein and carbohydrates) to feed the larvae, further weakening the future of the hive.[7]

Foraging honey bees use their crop to store nectar or water on the return trip to the hive. When preparing for a foraging or swarm flight, the crop is filled with honey from the comb to be utilized later as an energy source.[13] For longer, more consistent energy reserves, fat bodies on the dorsal and ventral surfaces of the inner abdomen are responsible for intermediate metabolism. This layer of cells provides a source of proteins and energy during long nonfeeding periods, such as overwintering.[7,14] These fat bodies also have been found to be the site for detoxification and vitellogenin (a female-specific phospholipoglycoprotein) production and are comparable to the mammalian liver and adipose tissues. These tissues appear to be more developed in younger worker bees than in foragers. Winter workers are much longer lived than summer workers and have well-developed fat bodies, optimal for overwintering.[15] In preparation for winter, apiarists must provide optimum conditions to promote well-developed fat bodies in fall brood. During the overwinter period, honey is the primary food source. Pollen is not available, except for that stored as bee bread (fermented product of pollen collected during foraging). The well-developed fat bodies of the winter workers provide the protein vitellogenin as the only source of amino acids, required to overwinter the queen and the colony. With appropriate assays and future work, it may be possible to use vitellogenin as an indicator of prewinter colony health.

Colony food shortage has been shown to affect behavioral development and social interactions of honey bees.[16,17] In starved colonies, behavioral development was accelerated; a significantly greater proportion of bees from starved colonies became foragers at significantly younger ages than in fed colonies. Colony nutritional status not only modulates the activity of bees already competent to forage but also affects long-term behavioral development.[16] Evaluation of social interactions in starved hives revealed a higher frequency of begging in starved bees compared with that of well-fed bees; this behavior increased exponentially as starvation became more severe, although no other behaviors differed consistently.[17] Pheromonal control also is affected in starving colonies. Queen mandibular pheromone (QMP) typically slows the transition from nursing to foraging. In times of starvation, QMP expression is altered and the pheromone exposure modifies the nutrient storage pathways and fat body gene expression. The QMP-treated workers in a starved hive survived much longer and had higher lipid levels than control bees.[18] Short-term larval starvation enabled bees, once adult, to shift to other fuels faster and showed an improved metabolic response and resilience to adult starvation.[19,20] Starved drone larvae resulted in smaller body size and abnormal wing size with changes more pronounced when starvation was later in larval development. Ejaculated semen volume, wing size asymmetry, and wing shape asymmetry, however, were not affected, preserving factors important for future reproduction.[21]

Honey bees cannot survive without honey. Starvation events may be difficult to predict, but with vigilant care these events may be curtailed by providing the hive with all the necessary tools to build stores successfully. A diagnosis of starvation almost always is made after the hive already has succumbed to starvation. Indications that starvation was the source of the colony demise include finding a cluster of bees dead on the floor of the hive between frames below where the cluster had been (**Fig. 1**); numerous deceased workers, each with nearly its entire body headfirst in the comb[22] (**Fig 2**); and dead bees attached to the comb at the site where the cluster had been. Honey stores at the site of the cluster, and possibly in the entire hive, are exhausted. It is possible, however, that the hive will have full frames of honey or other available supplemented foods that the bees did not consume or could not gain access to.

Prevention begins with attentive beekeeping and frequent hive inspections. During fall inspections, honey stores must be evaluated. Although amounts of honey required to overwinter vary by region, a good rule of thumb is that bees need at least 1 fully capped medium super (approximately 27 kg [60 lb] of honey, including what is stored in brood boxes) to survive the winter.[23] During winter inspections, hive lifts can be completed by lifting the entire hive gently from the back, pivoting the hive on the front edge. If the hive appears light, supplemental feeding may be facilitated using an in-hive feeder with a 2:1 sugar–to–water syrup ratio. Top feeders may not be accessible to the bees during cold days but may be useful in temperate winter climates. Similarly, Boardman entrance feeders unlikely are helpful because the bees cannot leave the cluster to access the syrup. Management practices may vary depending on geography, climate, and annual winter conditions.

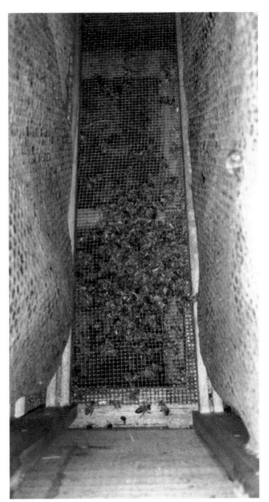

Fig. 1. A dead cluster following winter starvation. Notice the capped honey on either side of the cluster that was not accessed due to extended cold weather. (Picture courtesy of Dr. Jeff Applegate)

Queenless Laying Worker Colony

The queenless laying worker hive or laying worker colony (LCW) may well be 1 of the most frustrating conditions of the managed superorganism. Laying workers occur in the event when a queen dies and there is no brood of appropriate age to be selected and raised into a new queen. Typically, in a previously queenright hive that loses the queen, workers construct emergency queen cells from existing cells that contain diploid worker larvae that are less than 4 days old. If no brood of appropriate age is available from which to convert to emergency queen cells, the colony becomes help-lessly queenless, with a bleak future. If the colony cannot be reset with an accepted queen, the colony will die.

Routine hive inspections help identify this condition early and, if identified early, there may be a better chance of resolving the condition prior to occurrence of a

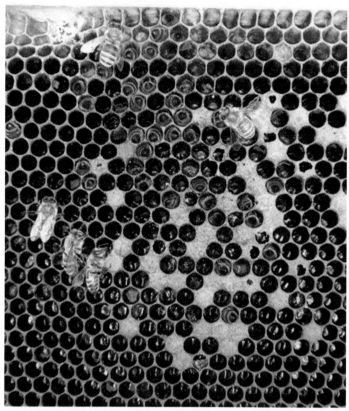

Fig. 2. A typical finding of bees buried headfirst in the comb adjacent to a cluster that has died from winter starvation. All the bees in this photograph are dead, the buried bees and the ones that died hanging on to the comb. Note the small number of brood cells that were being protected by the cluster. (Picture courtesy of Dr. Jeff Applegate)

doomed colony. The WLC condition usually occurs in the spring and early summer as queens are rearing colonies, although it also may occur at the start of a brand-new colony if the apiarist is unaware of the queen death or has not performed routine monitoring.

Upon inspection of the hive, a beekeeper or veterinarian may notice the characteristic unsettled loud buzz of a queenless colony.[24] Indications that the hive may be a laying worker colony include drone brood present where there was none 1 week prior, the brood pattern unusually scattered, eggs and brood found on the surface of frames and the walls of the hive,[25] and pathognomonic findings of multiple eggs haphazardly placed in cells (**Fig. 3**) and the presence of only drone brood (**Fig. 4**).[22,23,26] In cases of a WLC, unmated workers, having no stored sperm, lay unfertilized eggs, resulting in haploid brood and thus 100% drone offspring. This may be considered the colony's last-ditch effort to spread the previous queen's genetics in the face of a failing superorganism.

In a queenright colony, workers typically do not lay eggs; however, a small number can lay an occasional egg and may be responsible for the infrequent drone cell above a queen separator.[22,27,28] Without a queen, many workers start to experience ovarian

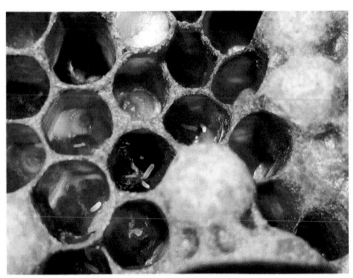

Fig. 3. In a laying worker hive, multiple eggs can be found in a single cell. Note the off-center and multiple eggs in single cells. (Photograph courtesy of Dr. Christophe Roy)

development due to the lack of the queen's pheromones responsible for worker ovarian suppression.[22] How quickly a honey bee colony begins to transition from queenless to a WLC is variable by subspecies. Egg-laying workers are much more common in Africanized honey bees than in European races.[29] European races tend to develop a laying worker environment after approximately 2 weeks, whereas some African honey bees are reported to develop laying workers after only 4 days to 8 days of queenlessness.[22,30,31] The earlier transition to laying workers in African races allows for laying worker even while a queen cell containing larvae is being

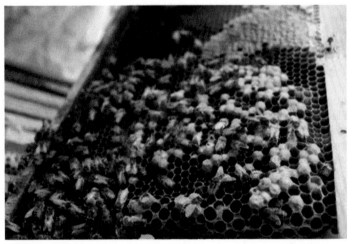

Fig. 4. Following the loss of a queen and initiation of a laying worker hive, only a drone brood is produced by the laying workers, usually in a scattered, unorganized pattern. (Picture courtesy of Dr. Nicolas Vidal-Naquet)

nurtured. The time needed for ovarian activation in European races is long enough, however, that the transition to a WLC is present only after there is no further chance that a replacement queen will emerge from the same colony.[29]

Endocrine suppression of worker ovarian development has been shown not only in *A mellifera* but also in *A cerana indica*.[32–34] Both species were evaluated under queen-right and queenless conditions, finding that they both had significantly higher amounts of certain pheromonal components that promote ovarian development and egg laying in laying workers compared with nonlaying workers.[34] Concordant with the development of worker ovaries, natural nursing behaviors and hive circadian rhythm are lost, due to the loss of the queen influence.[33] In studies involving Africanized honey bees in queenless colonies, hives fed candy that contained paprika resulted in precocious ovarian development in 15-day-old workers, whereas workers fed candy without paprika did not exhibit ovarian development as early. The result was explained by the fact that paprika contains high concentrations of bixin, a carotene rich in vitamin A.[35] Tyrosine, fed in royal jelly to larvae resulting in high brain levels of tyrosine, also has been linked to enhanced production of reproductive workers in queenless honey bee colonies.[36]

Management of a queenless laying worker hive can be difficult and, unfortunately, often unrewarding. If a new queen is not accepted to bring order to the colony, many beekeepers consider the WLC a lost cause and consider a shake-out of workers in front of another strong hive and restart the next season.[26] Requeening can be difficult because laying workers rarely accept a new queen. Astute observation and requeening before laying workers appear are likely best management. If the colony is not requeened successfully, it is doomed. Several methods have been reported with variable success:

- If another package or hive is available and doing well, move 1 frame to 2 frames of a capped/uncapped brood into the affected hive. Add a caged queen between frames, adjacent to the brood. This may result in the colony accepting the queen.[26]
- The chance of acceptance of a new queen may be improved if the brood frames are removed and replaced with an emerging worker brood. One report suggests that queen acceptance is returned to a satisfactory level if all combs are removed and the bees of the WLC are confined without food for 2 days. The brief starvation encourages the ovaries of the worker bees to return to normal.[22,37]
- In a report evaluating 3 methods of WLC management in 3 hives, there was variable success by method. Simply adding 2 combs of capped brood failed, and the colony was lost to poor hygiene and wax moths. A second method of adding a new mated queen and young workers also failed. A third method was reported successful. The hive was moved 200 m away from its original site in the evening; all bees and frames were removed; and frames were shaken out. The combs were tapped on a rock to dislodge eggs from the cells and the capped brood opened. The hive was returned to the original site. The foragers returned, but the laying workers remained on a tree near the shake site due to the inability to fly back to hive. The hive and workers were smoked and a mated queen and young workers were introduced and accepted.[38]
- One study evaluating 3 methods of requeening in hives that were queenless for 2 days or more showed good results, although this study did not report WLCs. In the first method, virgin queens, aged 3 days to 4 days, were introduced into 5-frame hives that had been dequeened 1 day, 2 days, 3 days, 4 days, 5 days, or 6 days previously. Duration of queenlessness significantly increased

acceptance, and direct introduction gave significantly greater success than artificial queen cell introduction (between 31% and 100% acceptance vs between 8% and 92% for direct introduction and cell introduction respectively, depending on the period of queenlessness).

In the second method, virgin and mated queens were introduced into 2-frame observation hives that had been dequeened 1 day, 2 days, 3 days, and 4 days previously. Mated queens resulted in a significantly higher probability of acceptance than virgin queens, for direct introduction versus artificial queen cells, and for longer queenless periods.

In the third method, mated queens were introduced into medium-sized hives (10 medium Langstroth frames) that had been queenless for 2 days using both the direct introduction and artificial cells. All queens were accepted.[39]

Hive Microenvironment

The internal hive environment is managed intensely. To maintain a stable environment, bees need to control temperature, ventilation, and humidity. The main focus usually is on brood temperature, although individual physiology and respiration, sanitation, and honey production result in waste products that need to be removed.

Overwintering can be a particularly challenging time for hive survival. Bees need protection from cold and wind. During the summer months, in addition to building honey stores, workers meticulously seal all the cracks and areas smaller than bee-space with propolis to eliminate drafts and solidify their fortress. To help prepare the hive for winter, medications and treatments, if indicated, and hive inspections should be initiated following summer honey harvest. Going into winter, each hive should have 1 frame to 2 frames of capped honey on either side of each brood box and a fullly capped super.[25] A strong hive needs approximately 27 kg (approximately 60 lb) of honey to get through the winter. Beekeepers must ensure that the colony has enough honey or carbohydrate resource to survive this challenging period; requirements may vary by region and winter intensity. By a month prior to winter, all treatments and frame rearrangement assistance should be concluded. A good windbreak should be provided, should a natural windbreak not be available. Straw bales may be used, but adequate ventilation must be maintained. Snow drift that blocks the entrance must be cleared because it impedes worker cleansing flights throughout the winter months.

Honey bees are heterothermic; during the winter months, the temperature inside the cluster allows the bees and potential larvae, if the queen is laying, to survive. If honey bee body temperature drops below approximately 39°F (approximately 4°C), a chill coma develops, resulting in muscular paralysis and potentially cessation of breathing mechanisms. As body temperature increases, workers become active at approximately 60°F (15.5°C) and do not fly until body temperature reaches 82°F (27.8°C).[26]

When the outside environmental temperature drops to 57°F (14°C), the bees begin to cluster around the queen and brood. The cluster usually begins in the center at the bottom of the hive. It then slowly migrates toward the top of the hive as resources are consumed. A cluster at the top of the hive in the winter is an indication that the hive is running out of resources. The cluster begins as a gathering of workers composed of an outer layer of tightly packed bees oriented with heads pointed toward the center. The inner area is packed less densely. The inner bees vibrate their wing muscles by repeated contractions to obtain thermal stability of the inner cluster with a temperature of approximately 95°F (35°C), the temperature required to raise brood; a brood fails to thrive below 90°F (32.2°C) and dies above 97°F (36.1°C). Wings are uncoupled from the flight muscles during the thermal muscle contractions to allow shivering without wing movements and prevent large air movements and wing damage while in the tight cluster. The bees in the outer shell of the cluster may be as cold as 45°F (7.2°C) but rotate through the middle of the cluster to warm up and have access to food. As the environmental temperature drops, the cluster becomes smaller and more compact, reducing the surface area and volume of the bees to keep warm. If extreme cold temperatures persist for a long time, the cluster may starve and die once the food within the cluster is spent. The persistent cold temperature does not allow the cluster to move to other areas of stored resources.

A chilled brood is a potential outcome of larvae that are not maintained at 95°F (35°C). If the cluster is not large enough to cover the brood, the exposed brood will die. A chilled brood is not exclusively a condition of winter. A brood can die from hypothermia in the spring build-up. This can occur through several avenues. The queen may be overzealous in the early season and lay more eggs than the workers can cover during cool times. A dead brood, in this instance, usually is found at the periphery of the brood patch (**Fig. 5**). Another cause may be iatrogenic where a beekeeper splits a hive early and an unexpected cool night kills exposed brood (**Fig. 6**). A brood that dies from hypothermia appears yellowish white to brown rather than pearly white; segmental margins may be tinged black. A capped chilled brood often has perforated cappings and appears similar to brood infected with American foulbrood but does not exhibit the signature ropey characteristics of AFB (**Fig. 7**).

Hive temperature not only is important during the cold season but also is regulated closely during the hot months. A relative constant temperature and humidity are maintained in the hive virtually all year long but may vary based on hive activity. Queen rearing hives have been show to drop their average internal temperature from greater than 93.2°F (34°C) to 82.4°F (28°C) during queen rearing, with the decrease greater in the front of the hive relative to the rear.[40] Temperatures above 97°F (36°C) are dangerous for the brood stock and cause death.[7] Hive cooling is necessary and appears achievable by the colony even when ambient outdoor temperatures well exceed this threshold. Cooling is the consequence of ventilation by workers fanning their wings

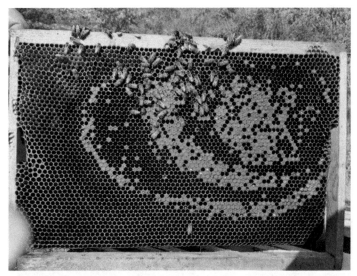

Fig. 5. The brood in this photo are dead following a chill event. Note the concentric rings where the periphery of the cluster could not keep the brood warm. (Photograph courtesy of Dr. Christophe Roy)

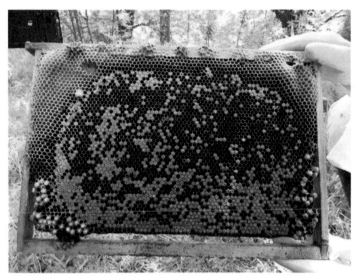

Fig. 6. The dead brood in this photo are due to an early spring hive split followed by an unexpected drop in temperature. The brood died due to the reduced number of workers available to cluster following the split. (Photograph courtesy of Dr. Christophe Roy)

inside the nest and at the entrance and also is due to evaporation of water spread in puddles on capped cells.[13] Bearding of bees at the entrance is an indicator of a potentially overheated hive. Access to water is essential for hive cooling of managed colonies.

Overheating occurs when hives are confined during hot weather and have limited to no access to water. Less likely in hobbyist or sideline hives, because water often is

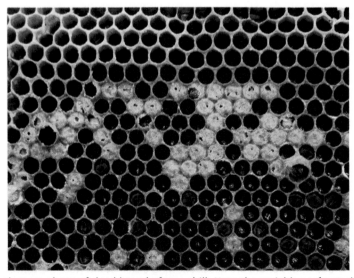

Fig. 7. A close-up photo of dead brood after a chill. Note the variably perforated caps and dead larvae. (Photograph courtesy of Dr. Christophe Roy)

easily available, this condition is overrepresented during commercial hive transport for honey flows or agricultural pollination services. Upon inspection of the hive, over-heated bees often are wet,[41] perhaps from regurgitated fluids in attempts to cool themselves, as has been reported..[22,42] When an overheated hive is opened, bees often seem disoriented and disperse by crawling rapidly in a disorderly manner and flutter their wings without flying. Overheating can be prevented by not confining bees on hot days and providing access to fresh water.

Humidity in the hive is a complex environmental variable. Accumulation of humidity is the result of exogenous conditions (outdoor environmental humidity) and endoge-nous effects, such as bees' metabolism and respiration, behavior, and nectar evapo-ration. Adequate ventilation is paramount to maintaining favorable humidity. Management may be completed via passive circulation or by active ventilation by workers fanning in the brood area. A balance must be struck between keeping the hive adequately humid without allowing condensation on the walls, brood, or honey comb. Although limited studies on hive humidity have been completed, 1 source re-ports relative humidity in healthy colonies tends to lie within the 40% to 60% range.[43] When 2 hives were tested side-by-side, 1 occupied and 2 empty, the empty hive re-flected roughly ambient humidity, although the physicality of the hive walls tended to be a bit of a buffer to high humidity. The occupied hive, however, remained at a rela-tively constant 65% to 70% humidity.[43] It is suggested that high humidity (>75%) may be detrimental to bees and brood favoring conditions, such as chalkbrood and dysen-tery. Strong colonies manage to minimize humidity variations better than weak col-onies. With future studies, it may be possible to use stability of relative humidity within a hive as a colony fitness indicator.

CLINICS CARE POINTS

- Starvation usually can be prevented by appropriate honey harvesting and properly preparing a colony for winter by providing enough stores to survive the winter months.
- A presumptive diagnosis of starvation can be made by necropsy.
- The laying worker hive often is considered a doomed hive and few techniques have been shown to recover a laying worker hive.

DISCLOSURE STATEMENT

The author has nothing to disclose.

REFERENCES

1. Kulhaneka K, Steinhauera N, Rennicha K, et al. A national survey of managed honey bee 2015–2016 annual colony losses in the USA. J Apicultural Res 2017;56(4):328–40.
2. Steinhauer N, Rennich K, Wilson M, et al. A national survey of managed honey bee 2012-2013 annual colony losses in the USA: results from the Bee Informed Partnership. J Apicultural Res 2014;53(1):1–18.
3. Lee K, Steinhauer N, Rennich K, et al. A national survey of managed honey bee 2013–2014 annual colony losses in the USA. Apidologie 2015;46:292–305.
4. Seitza N, Traynora K, Steinhauer N, et al. A national survey of managed honey bee 2014–2015 annual colony losses in the USA. J Apicultural Res 2015;54(4): 292–304.

5. Čápek J, Chlebo R. Summary of winter honey bee colony losses in Slovakia be-tween the years 2009 and 2015. Acta fytotechn zootechn 2016;19(1):22–4.

6. Huang Z. Honey Bee Nutrition. Am Bee J 2010;150(8):773–6.

7. Vidal-Naquet N. Honey bee veterinary medicine: Apis mellifera L. Sheffield, UK: 5m; 2015.

8. Shuel RW. The production of nectar and pollen. In: Graham JM, editor. The hive and the honey Bee. Hamilton, IL: Bookcrafters; 1992. p. 401–33.

9. Voorhies EC, Todd FE, Galbraith JK. Economic aspects of the bee industry, 555. Berkley, California: University of California College of Agriculture Bulletin; 1933. p. 1–117.

10. Kauffeld N, Everitt J, Taylor E. Honey bee problems in the Rio Grande Valley of Texas. Am Bee J 1976;116:220–2.

11. van Engelsdorp D, Meixner M. A historical review of managed honey bee popu-lation in Europe and the United States and the factors that may affect them. J Invertebr Pathol 2010;103:S80–95.

12. Riessberger U, Crailsheim K. Short-term effect of different weather conditions upon the behavior of forager and nurse honey bees (Apis mellifera carnica Poll-man). Apidologie 1997;28:411–26.

13. Winston ML. The biology of the Honey bee. Cambridge, MA: Harvard; 1987.

14. Arresse E, Soulages J. Insect fat body: energy metabolism, and regulation. Annu Rev Entomol 2010;55:207–25.

15. Imdorf A, Ruoff K, Fluri P. Le développement des colonies chez l'abeille mellifère. Berne: Station de recherche Agroscope Liebefeld-Posieux ALP; 2010.

16. Schulz D, Huang Z, Robinson G. Effects of colony food shortage on behavioral development in honey bees. Behav Ecol Sociobiol 1998;42:295–303.

17. Schulz D, Vermiglio M, Huang Z, et al. Effects of colony food shortage on social interactions in honey bee colonies. Insectes Sociaux 2002;49:50–5.

18. Fischer P, Grozinger C. Pheromonal regulation of starvation resistance in honey bee workers (Apis mellifera). Naturwissenschaften 2008;95:723–9.

19. Wang Y, Campbell J, Kaftanoglu O, et al. Larval starvation improves metabolic response to adult starvation in honey bees (Apis mellifera L.). J Exp Biol 2016; 219:960–8.

20. Wang Y, Kaftanoglu O, Brent C, et al. Starvation stress during larval development facilitates an adaptive response in adult worker honey bees (Apis mellifera L.). J Exp Biol 2016;219:949–59.

21. Szentgyörgyi H, Czekońska K, Tofilski A. The effects of starvation of honey bee larvae on reproductive quality and wing asymmetry of honey bee drones. J Apicultural Sci 2017;61(2):233–43.

22. Caldrone NW, Tucker KW. Variations, Abnormalities, and Noninfectious Diseases. In: Morse R, Flottum K, editors. Honey Bee Pests, Predators, and diseases. Ohio: A.I. Root Co; 1997. p. 401–23.

23. University of Georgia Honey Bee Program. Bees, beekeeping & protecting Polli-nators. Available at: https://bees.caes.uga.edu/bees-beekeeping-pollination/honey-bee-disorders.html. Accessed July 15, 2019.

24. Robles-Guerreroa A, Saucedo-Anayab T, González-Ramíreza E, et al. Analysis of a multiclass classification problem by Lasso Logistic Regression and Singular Value Decomposition to identify sound patterns in queenless bee colonies. Com-put Electronics Agric 2019;159:69–74.

25. Flottum K. The backyard beekeeper. Massachusetts: Quarry; 2010.

26. American Veterinary Medical Association. Honey Bees 101 for veterinarians 2019. Available at: https://www.avma.org/KB/Resources/Pages/Honey-Bees-101-Veterinarians.aspx. Accessed July 15, 2015.

27. Page RE Jr, Erickson EH Jr. Reproduction by worker honey bees (*Apis mellifera L.*). Behav Ecol Sociobiol 1988;23:117–26.

28. Visscher PK. A quantitative study of worker reproduction in honey bee colonies. Behav Ecol Sociobiol 1989;25:247–54.

29. Sommeijer MJ, Van der Blom J. Laying workers in Africanised honey bees, . Proceedings of the Section Experimental and Applied Entomology of The Netherlands Entomology Society (N.E.V.). Amsterdam, Netherlands: OMI, Utrecht; 1991.

30. Anderson RH. Some aspects of the biology of the Cape honey-bee. African Honey bees: taxonomy, biology and economic use. Pretoria: Apimondia; 1977.

31. Crewe RM, Hepburn HR, Moritz RF. Morphometric analysis of 2 southern African races of honey bee. Apidologie 1984;25:61–70.

32. Khajuria D, Dogra G. Endocrine control of oocyte maturation and vitellogenesis in the laying workers of the Indian hive bee (*Apis cerana indica Fab.*). Indian Bee J 1991;53(1–4):9–16.

33. Miller D III, Ratnieks F. The timing of worker reproduction and breakdown of policing behaviour in queenless honey bee (Apis mellifera L.). Insectes Sociaux 2001;48:178–84.

34. Tan K, Yang M, Wang Z, et al. The pheromones of laying workers in two honey bee sister species: *Apis cerana* and *Apis mellifera*. J Comp Physiol A 2012; 198:319–23.

35. Carneiro G, Chaud-Netto J, Arruda V, et al. Effect of paprika on the ovarian development of Africanized honey bee workers (*Apis mellifera L.*) in queenless colonies. Sociobiology 2008;52(3):567–77.

36. Matsuyama S, Nagao T, Sasaki K. Consumption of tyrosine in royal jelly increases brain levels of dopamine and tyramine and promotes transition from normal to reproductive workers in queenless honey bee colonies. Gen Comp Endocrinol 2015;211:1–8.

37. Orosi-Pal Z. [On laying workers] from an abstract in Bee World10, 1929. p. 134.

38. Kumar N, Kumar R. Successful management of a laying worker colony (*Apis cerana*). Am Bee J 1997;137(9):647.

39. Perez-Sato J, Kärcher M, Hughes W, et al. Direct introduction of mated and virgin queens using smoke: a method that gives almost 100% acceptance when hives have been queenless for 2 days or more. J Apicultural Res Bee World 2008;47(4): 243–50.

40. Chuda-Mickiewicz B, Prabucki J. Nest temperature of a queen rearing honey bee colony. Pszczeinicze zeszyty naukowe 1995;39(1):78–97.

41. Grimsley VM, Sadler G. A bridge between the North and the South. Am Bee J 1936;76:176–7.

42. Esch H. Foraging strategies in bees. Am Bee J 1976;116:568–9, 573.

43. Arnia remote hive monitoring (2017). Humidity in the Hive. Available at: https://www.arnia.co.uk/humidity-in-the-hive/. Accessed July 15, 2019.

Honey Bee Diagnostics

Don I. Hopkins[a],*, Jennifer J. Keller[b]

KEYWORDS

- Disease • Foulbrood • Nosema • Varroa • Chalkbrood • Sacbrood
- Small hive beetle • Tracheal mites

KEY POINTS

- American foulbrood is tentatively diagnosed based on clinical signs and field tests, but because of the consequences of a positive result, should be confirmed through a diagnostic laboratory.
- European foulbrood has various nonspecific clinical signs and often field diagnosis by ELISA is sufficient.
- Varroa mites are devastating to a colony and should be objectively quantified using a sugar shake or alcohol wash technique on a regular basis.
- Necropsy of a colony is an important diagnostic tool and should be completed systematically to best determine the cause of a dead hive.

 Video content accompanies this article at http://www.vetfood.theclinics.com.

INTRODUCTION

Before entering the apiary, light your smoker. Set the smoker aside and gather any tools and instruments for sample collection that you will use working in the hives. This should also include putting on your personal protection equipment. Once this is done check and make sure that the smoker that had been lit and set aside for several minutes is, in fact, still lit and working. This may seem elementary, but it should become appreciated as essential.

SIGHT, SOUND, SMELL, TASTE, AND TOUCH

How to use ours and the honey bee's primary senses needs to be understood. Veterinarians are trained to use all their sensory inputs when working with their patients. This is consistent in working with honey bees. The honey bee's primary sensory inputs seem to be sight, and smell in the form of communication pheromones. Honey bees are not particularly influenced by airborne sounds but do respond to vibrations

[a] North Carolina Department of Agriculture and Consumer Services, Plant Industry Division, NC, USA; [b] Department of Entomology and Plant Pathology, North Carolina State University, Campus Box 7613, Raleigh, NC 27695, USA
* Corresponding author. 381 Griffin Road, Snow Camp, NC 27349.
E-mail address: don.hopkins@ncagr.gov

Vet Clin Food Anim 37 (2021) 427–450
https://doi.org/10.1016/j.cvfa.2021.06.005
0749-0720/21/© 2021 Elsevier Inc. All rights reserved.

vetfood.theclinics.com

through a substrate, particularly in the nest structure. The handler should try to avoid unnecessary knocking and jarring of the nest. How taste and touch are used by the bees is fascinating to learn but is not as relevant to the manipulation of a colony as sight and smell (pheromone communication). The beekeeper, or a veterinarian performing a clinical examination, does need to have an awareness of how the honey bees respond to what they see. Sudden movements and certain colors are associated with colony threats. This is also true with odors that may stimulate an alarm response by the honey bees. Wearing lighter colors rather than darker colors is less threatening to the honey bees and therefore better for the beekeeper. One can use the honey bees' olfactory sense by properly using the smoker. It is an effective and safe way to direct much of the honey bees' behavior. Conversely the honey bees can use our sense of touch to effectively direct our behavior.

Before opening any of the hives check around the apiary to see if there are any external indicators of a problem. Look for crawling or twitching honey bees, dead immatures, dead adults, or marks and/or scratches on hives. Make note of any unusual odors.

When inspecting a colony, you need to get to the brood nest first. Generally, in a Langstroth hive the brood is toward the bottom of the hive. However, there are several circumstances that would cause the brood nest to be in the upper chamber. Such circumstances include, but are not limited to, the bees moving up through the food reserves, such as when overwintering or the colony has an extremely robust brood nest that expands above the normal lower hive cavity. A situation that is of concern regarding disease diagnosis is when cells are not appropriate for a queen to lay in causing her to move up into the area of comb that has not previously had any brood. This situation could be caused by debris or dead larvae (scale) remaining in the cell. This should indicate a greater rationale to investigate the abandoned brood area below.

In the brood nest, examine enough frames to evaluate all stages of a full brood cycle. You should see eggs; developing larva; and capped brood, which contains the pupal stage of the bees. In all castes, the eggs exist for about 3 days. In the case of workers and drones the feeding or larval stage exists for around 6 days. The capped stage in workers is 12 days and for drones it is 3 days longer. In the development of queens, the larval and pupal stages are accelerated; the feeding stage lasts only about 5 days and the capped stage lasts about 8 days.

AMERICAN FOULBROOD (*PAENIBACILLUS LARVAE*)

American foulbrood (AFB) is a bacterial disease that infects larvae at a very young point in its development. The effects of the disease are expressed at a specific age, just after encapsulation where the prepupa dies in the cell. The appearance of the capped brood is the most relevant in the case of AFB. Healthy brood should appear even and solid and any deviation from this needs to be investigated. If the cappings are perforated, that is a strong indicator that the pupae are not healthy. In addition, if the caps are sunken or greasy looking, these may be indicators of AFB (**Fig. 1**).

Associated with AFB there is often a peculiar odor. It has been compared with thrush hoof smell or animal hide gluepot odor. This odor is often noted before or immediately on opening the hive. Once in the brood nest find a brood frame that looks suspicious and investigate individual cells (**Fig. 2**). With a toothpick or matchstick, probe a cell, stir contents, and slowly draw it out (**Fig. 3**). If the content is viscous, it will string out the distance equal to five or more cells and then snap back, an indication of AFB. This is the vegetative stage of AFB as it sporulates in the remains of the prepupa.

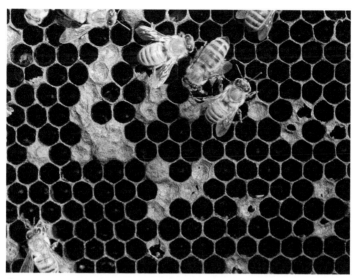

Fig. 1. Perforated cell cappings indicating possible brood disease.

Paenibacillus larvae is a spore-forming bacteria. As the material desiccates, the remnants in the cell of the comb adhere tightly to the cell wall and form what is called a scale. The scales sit just below the surface of the comb (**Fig. 4**). The comb is angled so that looking at the comb straight on, the scale is not visible. Therefore, it is important to slightly angle the frame so that the top of the comb is closer to the viewer than the bottom (**Fig. 5**). Looking down the top face of the comb the scales are apparent on the lower walls of each cell. A simple examination of the comb is done with a UV light

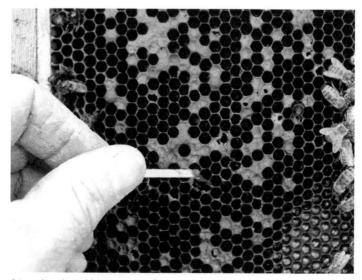

Fig. 2. Probing discolored larva to test for AFB.

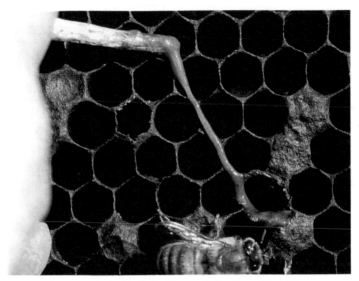

Fig. 3. Demonstrating rope test of infected larva distinctive with AFB.

under which the scale fluoresce (**Figs. 6** and **7**). Each scale contains approximately 2.5 billion spores.

Field and Laboratory Diagnostics

In addition to the matchstick test, an enzyme-linked immunosorbent assay (ELISA) test is available for AFB and also one for European foulbrood (EFB) that is used to corroborate what is observed. Swabs are taken from apparently infected cells; the swab is placed in the solution that comes with the package. Drops are then placed

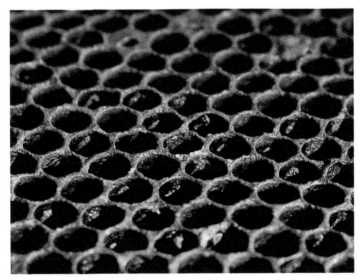

Fig. 4. Scales sitting just below surface of the comb.

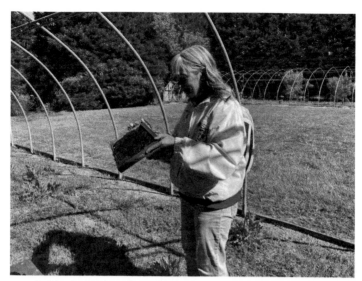

Fig. 5. How to hold a brood frame to best view AFB scale.

onto the strip. There are two letters on the stick: T indicates test and C indicates control. If it tests positive, two distinct lines appear. If only one appears at the letter C, that is considered a negative. If neither line appears the test is invalid (**Fig. 8**). This kit may be used as a tool to support the corroborating evidence in determining a diagnosis; it should not supplant the knowledge and skills of the diagnostician.

Sampling and Shipping

When needing to collect a sample to send to a diagnostic laboratory, the best sampling method is to cut a small section of comb containing several of the infected cells. Wrap the section of comb in newspaper, paper towel, or other permeable material. Do

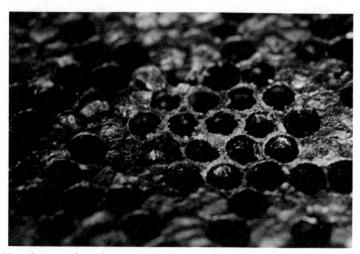

Fig. 6. AFB scale in comb under normal light.

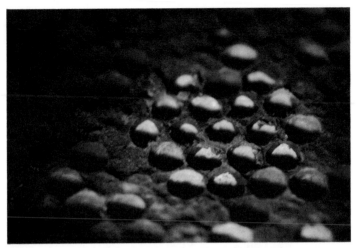

Fig. 7. AFB scale in comb under UV light (same scale as **Fig. 6**).

not wrap in plastic. A section of comb is preferable because it yields more information, but a swab of infected larvae is used as an alternative technique. If testing for AFB, a swab could be used directly for preparing a slide to test for Brownian motion or could be cultured. In the case of EFB (discussed later), a swab may not prove as useful. The swab should also be wrapped in paper before shipping. Check with the laboratory before collecting the sample to verify their sampling protocol and criteria for shipping. Depending on what is being tested, time may be a critical factor. When a brood sample is received, either a smear or preferably a section of infected comb, it is checked for the presence of *P larvae* using the hanging drop method as described by the US Department of Agriculture ARS Handbook Diagnosis of Honey Bee Diseases.[1] A smear is placed on a cover glass and heat fixed under a heat lamp. It is then stained

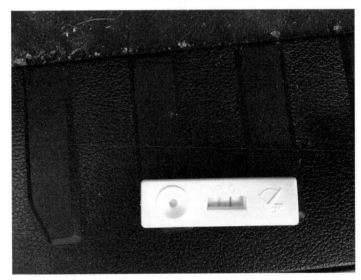

Fig. 8. ELISA test strip indicating a positive test.

with carbol fuchsin. After the stain has been allowed to fully penetrate the sample, the excess is rinsed with water. While still wet, the cover glass is inverted onto a microscope slide that has been smeared with a layer of immersion oil. The slide is gently blotted with bibulous paper and then observed under the microscope. The *P larvae* spores exhibit Brownian motion in the water suspended on the oil (**Fig. 9**, Video 1). If further verification is needed AFB may also be cultured on a medium of brain-heart infusion.[1]

EUROPEAN FOULBROOD (*MELISSOCOCCUS PLUTONIUS*)

EFB, like AFB, is a bacterial disease. However, EFB is not as serious to the colony as AFB because it is not a spore-forming bacteria, which means it is not as contagious and can be cleared up. The causative organism is *Melissococcus plutonius*, which generally affects the larval stage. Unlike AFB, which consistently affects the larvae at a specific development stage, EFB is much less consistent. The effect of the organism on the larva is generally apparent before it reaches the capped stage. The result is a larva that appears different from the normal pearly white. Infected larva appear yellow to brown in color. At this stage, the tracheal system may appear as a series of white lines on the darkened larva (**Fig. 10**). The larva may possibly be misshapen, and not necessarily in any set position in the cell (**Fig. 11**).

Probing a diseased larva helps determine what the cause might be. With EFB, when probing an infected cell, the larva are somewhat viscous, but do not have the same stringiness that is typical with AFB. The infected larva do not string out much more than the width of a cell, whereas with AFB it strings out about one inch (~2.5 cm). If the disease is far enough along to where the larva has desiccated and a scale has formed on the bottom of the cell walls, it is easily removed, unlike AFB where the scales adhere to the cell wall and are difficult to dislodge.

Generally, there is a pronounced, sharp, sour odor associated with this brood disease, but the odor can vary from case to case. *Paenibacillus alvei* is a secondary bacterium that is often associated with *M plutonius*.[2] When *P alvei* is cultured it produces a

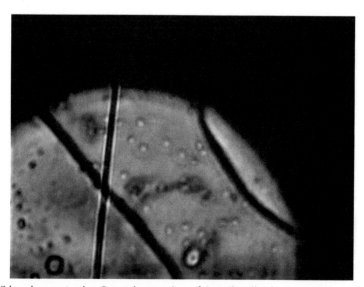

Fig. 9. Video demonstrating Brownian motion of *Paenibacillus larvae* spores.

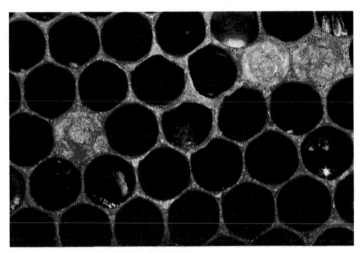

Fig. 10. Infected larva with visible tracheal tubes.

strong unpleasant odor. The presence of secondary bacteria may account for the variation of odors observed. Often, the odor is detected as soon as the hive is opened by the beekeeper.

Field and Laboratory Diagnostics

An ELISA test is also available for EFB and the same steps are followed as were described in the section on AFB. For EFB, this kit is a much more useful tool for a quick diagnosis because this disease is easy to confuse in the field with other maladies, such as parasitic mite syndrome (PMS), AFB, sacbrood, starvation, and several others. This test should easily differentiate EFB from the others.

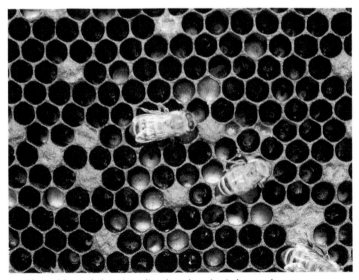

Fig. 11. EFB-infected brood showing discolored and misshapen larvae.

M plutonius is cultured in the laboratory using Bailey medium in anaerobic environment.[1] Although it may be done, it is difficult to isolate from other bacteria that are associated with EFB and culturing takes at least 96 hours to obtain results. The ELISA test may be a more reasonable option of detection to determine what course of action should be implemented.

The preferred method of sampling and shipping for EFB is a small section of comb. See the section on AFB for further explanation.

SACBROOD

Sacbrood is a viral brood disease affecting honey bee larvae and could be mistaken for AFB or EFB. Symptoms of sacbrood involve a less than solid brood pattern that in severe cases may appear spotty. In an area of capped brood there will be cells that are prematurely uncapped by the adults. Inside the individual cell is an infected larva that appears brown in color and generally is extended the length of the cell. It is commonly described as appearing canoe shaped, because the head tends to lift off from the base of the cell (**Fig. 12**). When probing the cell, the entire larvae can be pulled out and looks like a hanging sac of liquid (**Fig. 13**). The cuticle is toughened and that is why the liquid remains in the sac.

Because it is a virus, and there is more awareness of the ability of mites to vector the viruses, controlling for varroa mites may help in preventing its spread. Because of the initial appearance in the comb, the greatest concern about sacbrood is to be sure it is not one of the more serious brood diseases. Once determined to be sacbrood, using the aforementioned observations closely monitor the situation, but not much action is necessary except in extreme cases. If the symptoms persist after a brood cycle, action may be necessary, such as requeening. Of the dozens of viruses found in honey bee colonies, this is one of several that are screened for using polymerase chain reaction, but it is often not necessary because the symptoms typically clear up on their own.

CHALKBROOD (*ASCOSPHAERA APIS*)

Chalkbrood is a common brood disease caused by a fungus, *Ascosphaera apis*. It affects the larvae just after it stretches out and is ready to encapsulate. This is probably

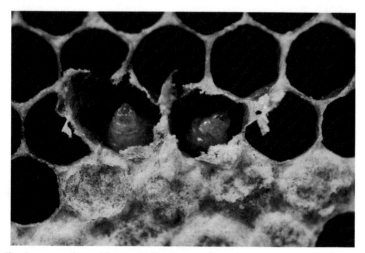

Fig. 12. Classic canoe-shaped larvae indicating sac brood.

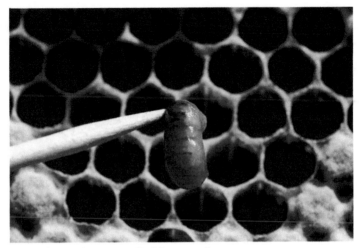

Fig. 13. Larva in the saclike state pulled from a cell.

the simplest to detect and the simplest to differentiate from the other brood diseases. The larvae gets a white chalky appearance or sometimes they may turn gray or black depending on whether there are fruiting bodies present.[3] These affected larvae are called "mummies." They have the texture and consistency of a piece of chalk, thus the name chalkbrood (**Fig. 14**). A heavily infected frame when shaken releases the hardened larvae. An observant beekeeper, inspector, or veterinarian might notice some of these mummies in front of the hive or possibly on the bottom board because the honey bees try to clean out the affected larvae. This is perhaps the easiest disease to identify in the field because the mummified larvae are pathognomonic. Some honey

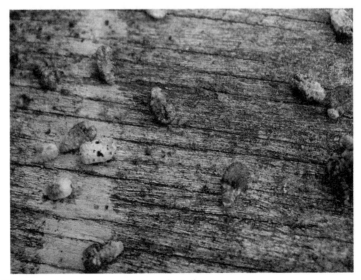

Fig. 14. Chalkbrood mummies on bottom board.

bees are more hygienic than others and do a better job of cleaning out the dead (**Fig. 15**).

Although not considered a serious disease, chalkbrood can weaken a colony to the point of making it nonproductive. It usually occurs in the spring when there are cool and damp conditions. Like EFB, chalkbrood is considered a stress-related disease where external factors compete with the bees' attention. By adjusting environmental conditions, the honey bees may have a chance to catch up.

VARROA MITES (*VARROA DESTRUCTOR*)

The greatest concern facing beekeepers today is the varroa mite, *Varroa destructor*. PMS is a common problem associated with high levels of mites leading to the decline of the adult honey bee population within a colony. Varroa mites may be found at every developmental stage of the bee except the egg. Although large, mites obscure themselves, hiding in cells and among adult bees, making them difficult to detect during a routine inspection.

Aside from finding the actual mites, an apparent symptom of a mite problem is a spotty brood pattern on a capped brood frame. This is similar to that found with EFB, sacbrood, and even AFB to some extent. Cappings may be perforated or partially open but do not appear sunken. By probing these cells, healthy, pearly white, pupae are found beneath the cappings, unlike with foulbrood where the larva are brown or yellow in color. Also lacking is the distinctive odor usually found with AFB and EFB. Often a spotty brood pattern is attributed to an inferior queen; however, further inspection to find an egg frame may reveal a healthy queen with a good egg laying pattern. At this point it is obvious the queen is laying consistently, but the larvae and pupae are not developing at the same rate, thus leading to population decline.

Bald-headed brood, open cells with partially developed pupae, is a condition also associated with PMS. In the presence of high mite levels, adult workers open some of the capped cells and investigate the pupae (**Fig. 16**). Occasionally the pupae are partially removed, with remnants of pupae remaining in the cell. The remains are

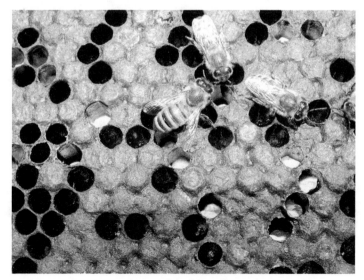

Fig. 15. Brood frame showing evidence of chalkbrood mummies in cells.

usually white as opposed to yellow or brown like the other brood diseases. There are other causes for bald-headed brood, such as wax moths that burrow in the comb and cause damage.

There are a few other signs to look for to help confirm the diagnosis of mite problems. Workers appearing smaller than normal with deformed wings is a strong indication of high levels of mites (**Fig. 17**). These bees will never be able to fly so crawling bees may be seen in front of the hive. At the entrance of the hive there might be visible signs of the white immature bees being carried out the front.

Knowing the history of colony management is helpful. The next step is to perform a sugar shake or alcohol wash to determine the mite infestation level. Depending on findings, action may be warranted.

Alcohol Wash

One method for determining mite infestation is the alcohol wash. The purpose of an alcohol wash is to determine the number of mites relative to the number of bees in a hive. Mites are primarily found in the capped brood or pupal stage of bees, and secondarily (in their phoretic stage) traveling on the adult bees. It is not easy to sample the brood. Instead, sampling the attendant adult bees can give a reasonable estimate of the mite population in the colony. The adults with the highest portion of mites will be the nurse bees or recently emerged bees and this is the area that should be sampled. A suitable frame for sampling is one that has a mix of maturing larvae and capped pupae with attendant adult bees. Bees sampled from a honey frame give a false read.

After selecting the frame, look for the queen so she is not included in the sample. Next, collect approximately 300 bees from the frame. Adult bees are collected by shaking the bees off the frame into a collection pan. Some of the bees may fly off,

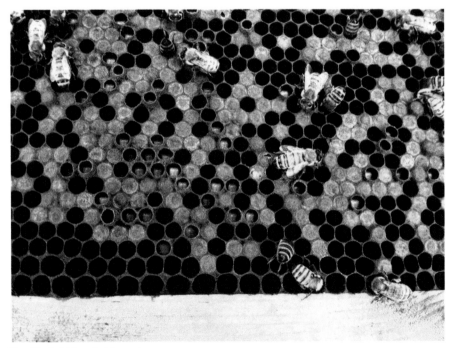

Fig. 16. Bald-headed brood.

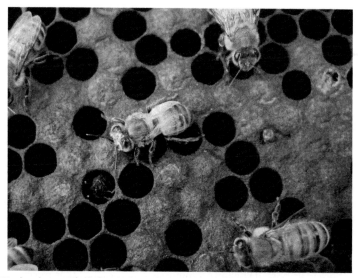

Fig. 17. Worker bee with deformed wing virus vectored by the varroa mite.

but that is not a problem. Knock remaining bees into one corner of the pan and then scoop enough bees to fill a half a cup measure. A half cup of bees is about 300 bees. That half cup of bees is placed into a sample jar containing 70% alcohol.

The bees are shaken vigorously in the jar with alcohol then poured through an eight-mesh sieve (**Fig. 18**) with a finer filter below to collect the mites. The bees remain above the sieve and mites fall through. These bees can then be rewashed and rinsed several times through the eight-mesh sieve until no further mites are collected (**Fig. 19**). The mites are then counted, and the bees are also counted, which gives a

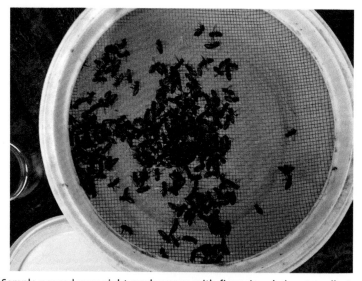

Fig. 18. Sample poured over eight-mesh screen with finer sieve below to collect mites.

precise mite to bee ratio. The critical aspect of this procedure is to collect a sample from a suitable frame.

Sugar Shake

The sugar shake is an alternative method of checking for mites. One advantage with this method is the sugar-coated bees are returned to their colony alive. The advantage of the alcohol wash over the sugar shake is that it is more precise because the actual number of bees is counted instead of estimated. The steps used to collect bees for an alcohol wash are also used here. It is important to choose a frame from the brood nest with maturing larvae and some recently capped brood. After checking that the queen is not present, the adult bees are knocked off into a collecting tub and a half-cup scoop of bees then removed and placed into the shaking container. It is nothing more than a wide-mouth jar with an eight-mesh screen for a lid. After the screen is placed on top, trapping the bees in the jar, add two heaping tablespoons of dry powdered sugar to the top and sift through the screen onto the bees. Gently shake to ensure bees are coated. Set aside and allow about 5 minutes for the bees to become completely coated with the sugar. The sugar acts as a slight irritant to the honey bees causing them to groom more vigorously and also interferes with the mite's ability to adhere to its host. If shaken prematurely, many of the mites may not have had time to dislodge. If too much time passes, the sugar does not maintain its powdery consistency, which may give a false read. At this point the bees are shaken over any light-colored surface (**Fig. 20**). The mites fall through the screen while the bees remain in the jar. A white bucket lid with a shallow amount of water is helpful. The water dissolves the sugar and allows the mites to float on the surface tension of the water. The mites are easy to see and count (**Fig. 21**). After several good strong shakes the number of mites can be counted. Because there are approximately 300 honey bees in a half-cup sample, the number of mites collected divided by three gives a rough percentage of mites to bees. This information helps determine if there is a mite problem in this colony. Knowing the mite to bee ratio is critical in determining the health of the colony.

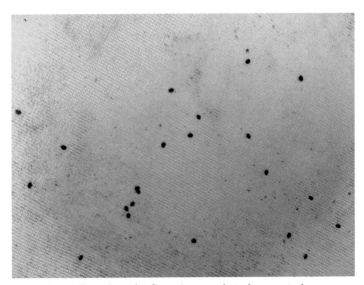

Fig. 19. Varroa mites collected on the finer sieve ready to be counted.

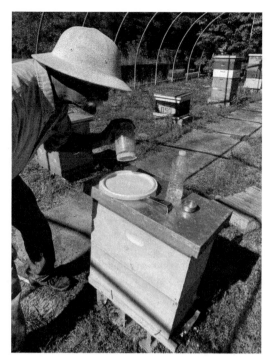

Fig. 20. Testing a hive for varroa mites using the sugar-shake method.

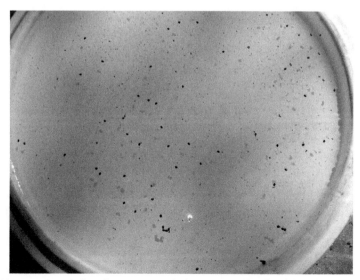

Fig. 21. Varroa mites shaken from a sugar shake jar into a bucket lid with water.

It is important to remember when using this technique, it is necessary to collect bees of the right age and to use dry powdered sugar. The bees must be young nurse bees collected from the brood nest. If foragers are sampled the results will not be a true mite count.

Other Monitoring Methods

Crude indication of mite levels is established by the use of a sticky board on the bottom board or checking a small sample of burr comb, which frequently contains drone brood. A sticky board is not quantitative like the alcohol or sugar shake methods. The sticky board is a thin, stiff board, approximately the same size as a bottom board with a thin layer of petroleum jelly applied or other sticky/jelly-like substance, such as cooking spray. Sticky boards are placed under an eight-mesh screened bottom board and used to monitor the natural mite drop over a 24-hour period. After this time, the boards are removed, and the mites may be counted. This determines if mites are present in the colony, but it does not consider the size of the colony, so it is difficult to determine an accurate percentage of mite infestation. Another quick test is to look at a section of drone brood or piece of burr comb and inspect for mites in the cells. These methods are screening tools; should mites be detected with either of these screening tests, it is good practice to evaluate further using either the alcohol or sugar shake method.

TRACHEAL MITES (ACARAPIS WOODI)

The tracheal mite is an internal parasite that infests the tracheal tubes of the adult honey bee. Bees that are crawling outside the hive, particularly after a cold spell, may be infested with tracheal mites. This syndrome is most likely to be expressed in late winter or early spring. Dissection is necessary for confirmation.

Unlike with *Varroa*, older worker bees are more likely to be infested. There is a greater likelihood that these organisms will have had time to move into and reproduce in the trachea of the bee. Collecting those bees that are crawling outside the hive has a greater probability of revealing the infestation. This sample could be supplemented with bees from the outer perimeter of the colony, such as those on the inner cover. A minimum of 50 bees should be collected in 70% alcohol. The standard number to dissect is 25, but it is a good idea to have extra to ensure there are at least 25 good samples to examine under the microscope.

Laboratory Diagnostics

At the laboratory the bees are sectioned by removing the head and first pair of legs; this is a natural breakpoint. With a sharp scalpel or razor blade cut a 2-mm cross-section from the anterior end of the thorax (**Fig. 22**). These thoracic disks contain a significant amount of muscle tissue and the first pair or primary pair of tracheal tubes. Tracheal mites tend to gravitate to this area of the bee. These are put into a 5% to 10% solution of KOH for approximately 24 hours, which dissolves the muscle tissue leaving only the trachea.[1] During microscopic examination at ×100 power, any dark blotches in the tracheal tubes may be evidence of either scarring or the actual mites living in the tracheal lumen (**Fig. 23**). The trachea appears as transparent spiral tubules when no mites are present (**Fig. 24**).

Another method is the use of 85% lactic acid instead of KOH. The lactic acid softens the muscle tissue rapidly and the tissue is removed from the chitinous exoskeleton so the trachea is teased out.[1]

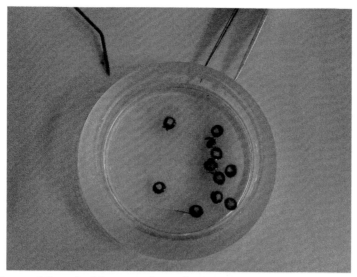

Fig. 22. Prepared thoracic disks to test for tracheal mites.

NOSEMA (*NOSEMA* SP)

Nosema is a microsporidian that infects the midgut of the adult honey bee and is often associated with honey bee dysentery. Two commonly noted symptoms are spotting on the hive (**Fig. 25**) and bees crawling at the entrance of the hive. If either is noticed further sampling may be performed. Nosema is one of the easier conditions to sample and view under a microscope. A minimum of 50 adult bees should be collected. Only 30 bees are tested in the laboratory, but it is a good idea to collect extra. Samples should be taken from older bees and preserved in 70% alcohol until processed in

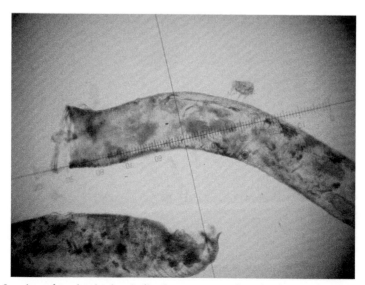

Fig. 23. Scarring of tracheal tubes indicating presence of tracheal mites (×100 power).

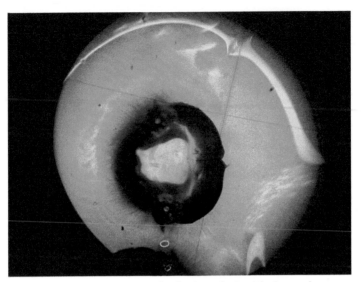

Fig. 24. Thoracic disk demonstrating tracheal tubes of a healthy honey bee.

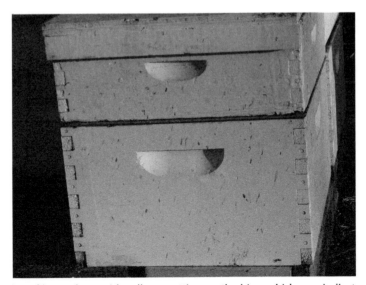

Fig. 25. Hive of honey bees with yellow spotting on the hive, which may indicate nosema.

the laboratory. Methods of collecting samples include live honey bees, bees on dry ice, or bees saturated in alcohol and drained. It is important to check with the receiving laboratory before sampling to confirm proper collecting and shipping protocols.

Laboratory Diagnostics

Remove the abdomen of 30 older honey bees and macerate in 30 mL of water using a mortar and pestle. An alternative is to put the abdomens in a plastic sandwich bag with the water and use a rolling pin to crush the contents.[1] Place one drop of the solution onto a microscope slide and view at ×400 power (**Fig. 26**).

This method determines the presence of nosema spores using a subjective score based on low, moderate, or high counts. A more precise method incorporates the use of a hemocytometer to determine the number of spores per bee.[1] These methods do not differentiate between the species of *Nosema apis* or the more prevalent *Nosema ceranae*.

With *N apis*, knowing the exact spore count is useful in determining the treatment protocol. The threshold for treatment is a million spores per bee. However, now that *N ceranae* seems to be displacing *N apis*, exact counts are not as important, because the treatment thresholds for *N ceranae* are indeterminate. There is an antimicrobial effective for treating *N apis*, but there is debate as to its efficacy in treating *N ceranae*.

SMALL HIVE BEETLE (*AETHINA TUMIDA*)

The small hive beetle is a common pest of honey bees in warm, humid climates. The beetles are easily noticed and often spotted when first opening a hive. They may be seen in a top feeder, just beneath the inner cover, or in between boxes during a routine inspection. They appear as quick moving black beetles about the size of a lady beetle (ladybug; Family: Coccinellidae) but flatter in appearance. The two distinguishing characteristics are the shield-shaped thorax and the club-shaped antennae (**Fig. 27**).

The beetles tend to congregate in the outer perimeter of the colony nest. Depending on the size of the nest and the environmental conditions, this may be on the uppermost

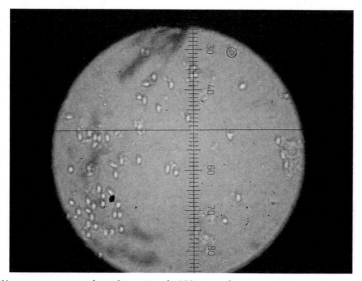

Fig. 26. Nosema spores under microscope (×400 power).

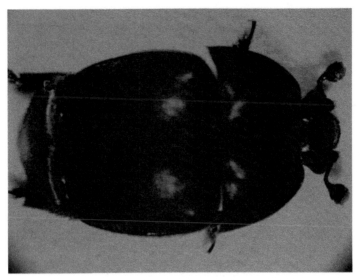

Fig. 27. Small hive beetle easily recognized by the club-shaped antennae and shield-shaped thorax.

part of the hive or the bottom portion of the hive. Quantifying their impact on a colony is difficult, particularly if only adult beetles are present. The beetle larvae, however, can severely impact a colony.

It is important to detect problems and find solutions early when dealing with small hive beetles. One sign to be aware of is an odor like rotting or fermenting fruit. This is a sign beetle larvae are doing physical damage to the colony. Further inspection of each frame is necessary to locate the specific area of outbreak. At early stages, larvae are small, feed inside individual cells, and may not be obvious. As the larvae grow, they are more easily seen because they leave the cells (**Fig. 28**). A second

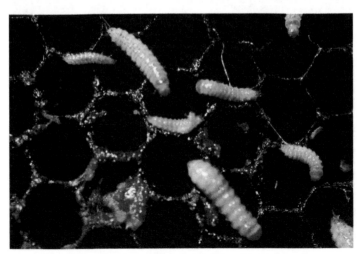

Fig. 28. Larvae of small hive beetle crawling on surface of brood comb.

indication may be noticed in the area where the pollen is stored. Under normal conditions, the bees pack the pollen, so the surface of each cell is smooth. In the presence of beetle larvae, the pollen is no longer smooth, but percolates out from the cells, and appears powdery. Often this powder may be noticed on the bottom board or at the entrance of the hive. If these conditions are caught early, it is possible to remove the affected frames and save the remaining part of the colony. If damage is too great, the bees will not be able to overcome the infestation and will eventually abscond.

NECROPSY

When a colony of dead bees is discovered in an apiary, it is difficult to determine the exact cause for its ultimate demise; however, information is gleaned by any evidence that is left in the hive, particularly if the beekeeper has not cleaned the equipment. Therefore, it is useful to examine the remains, once again using all senses. A conversation with the beekeeper about the history and management is also useful.

Before opening the hive, make some initial observations.

Is there any noticeable odor?
- A general dead bee smell indicates the bees died in the hive.
- A more specific odor, such as that described for AFB or EFB, could indicate a bacterial brood disease.
- A chemical smell might indicate a pesticide issue.
- A rotting or fermenting fruit smell (rotten oranges) could indicate a small hive beetle problem.

Visual clues may be observed outside the hive before inspecting.
- Signs of yellow streaking on the outside of the hive is a sign of dysentery, possibly *Nosema*.
- Recent scratches or chewed wood on the corners, or clumps of chewed bee bodies suggest small mammal predation, such as raccoon, possum, or skunk. Major damage could be a bear.

Check the immediate area in front of the hive for dead or dying bees, which could be an indication of pesticide, starvation, mite depredation, or robbing.
- Are there piles of bees at the entrance? This could indicate pesticide, robbing from another colony, or starvation.
- Are there any surviving bees crawling or twitching around the hive? This may be caused by tracheal mites, pesticides, starvation, or a virus.
- What age are the dead? Adults, pupae, larvae? If adults, it is more likely to be pesticide (possibly viral). If there are pupae and larvae, it is more likely to be another organism, such as varroa mites or small hive beetle, or starvation.

At this point, if nothing is obvious, begin to disassemble the hive taking time for observations along the way. As boxes are removed, notice if the boxes are heavy or light. Also look for dead bees where the cluster should have been and any sign of pests.

While disassembling the hive:
- If it is heavy, it is obvious it did not die directly from starvation and needs further investigation.
- If it is light, or no food, it is possible it died of starvation or the honey was robbed by other bees.
- Is there a ball of dead bees? Are they head first, tails out in the cells of the honey frames? This is an indication that the colony died of starvation.
- Working toward the center of where the brood nest should be, look for any sign of brood disease, such as perforated cappings or presence of scale. This could be

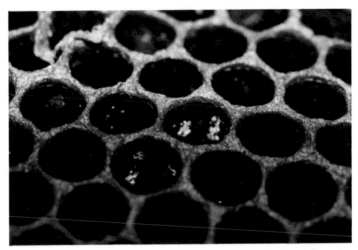

Fig. 29. Excrements deposited on upper cell walls from previous mite infestation.

AFB or EFB. See the section on these diseases for further description. If AFB is suspected, isolate the hive from the yard until confirmed. If determined positive, it may be necessary to destroy the equipment according to state regulations.

- Check capped brood for varroa mites by probing cells and examining pupae and check for mite excrement in these cells (tiny white crystals on top walls of the cell) (**Fig. 29**).
- While looking at the darker brood comb, look for wax moth tunnels, and for beetle grubs. This is common to find in abandoned hives, but these are usually a result of other events, often not the cause of its demise.
- Look for evidence of queen events. Evidence may be indicated by presence of used queen cells, multiple eggs in cells, or all drone brood (**Fig. 30**). An

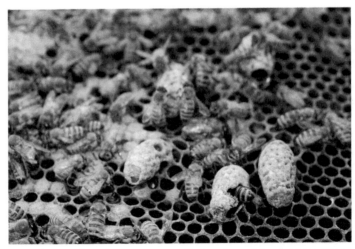

Fig. 30. Emerged, capped, and open queen cells showing evidence of recent queen event.

unsuccessful queen event could be the cause of the colony dwindling to a point where it could no longer survive.

- When all frames have been inspected, remove the bottom box to examine the bottom board. What may appear as useless debris on the bottom board may have useful clues. Before scraping off debris, examine closely.
- A pile of dead bees inside the hive most likely indicates starvation. Other possibilities include pesticides, robbing, or suffocation on rare occasions.
- A thick layer of wax cappings on the bottom board indicates the hive was robbed.
- If the colony had high numbers of varroa mites, they will be found on the bottom board under all other debris. If many mites are found, PMS could have been the primary problem.
- Look for beetle grubs and any other organisms in the debris on the bottom board. If there is a layer of wax cappings, the beetles will be hiding underneath.

As this is being done, the beekeeper is likely to recall a more detailed history of the hive management.

SUMMARY

Many diseases and pests have been discussed in this article, and it is important for the beekeeper and the veterinarian to be able to distinguish the different symptoms for each. This may be a valuable tool because not all the diseases are equally alarming. There are three main ones that beekeepers and veterinarians need to be aware of. AFB and varroa mites are the greatest concern for beekeepers; varroa because of their prevalence and potential damage, and AFB because of its devastating impact to a colony and contagion in an apiary. Both are fairly easy to identify and sample for, to verify their presence (or absence). EFB is the other brood disease that may be a problem and is the hardest to differentiate. A veterinarian should be able to segregate EFB from the other maladies before use of antibiotics. It is helpful to be able to identify all the other diseases described if only to rule them out during diagnosis, but generally, these do not decimate an apiary. It is important to be observant and take care of problem hives early before opportunistic pests, such as the small hive beetle and the wax moth, cause a much larger problem. Colonies need to be healthy to survive and prosper.

CLINICS CARE POINTS

- Proper use of a smoker can aid the veterinarian performing clinical examinations on honey bee colonies.
- Veterinarians are most often called on to diagnose the bacterial diseases, AFB and EFB, but should be knowledgeable on the other honey bee diseases to arrive at the correct diagnosis.
- EFB is particularly challenging to diagnose, but the field ELISA test kit can help to quickly rule in or out the diagnosis.
- EFB is treated with antibiotics and the colony may recover, but because AFB is extremely contagious it should be eliminated from an apiary.
- Problems caused by varroa mites is the most common problem in honey bee colonies, but may also be the easiest to diagnose when mite levels are high.

DISCLOSURE

The authors have nothing to disclose.

SUPPLEMENTARY DATA

Supplementary data related to this article can be found online at https://doi.org/10.1016/j.cvfa.2021.06.005.

REFERENCES

1. Shimanuki H, Knox D. Diagnosis of honey bee diseases. U.S. Department of Agriculture; 2000. Agriculture Handbook No. AH-690.
2. Shimanuki H. Bacteria. In: Morse RA, Flottum K, editors. honey bee pests, predators and diseases. 3rd edition. Medina (OH): Al Root Company; 1997. p. 35–55.
3. Gilliam M, Vandenberg JD. Fungi. In: Morse RA, Flottum K, editors. Honey bee pests, predators and diseases. 3rd edition. Medina (OH): Al Root Company; 1997. p. 81–110.

Registered Medicinal Products for Use in Honey Bees in the United States and Canada

Tracy S. Farone, BS, DVM

KEYWORDS

- Honey bee antibiotics • Veterinary honey bee medications • Antibiotic resistance
- Veterinary feed directive (VFD)

KEY POINTS

- A brief history of the origins of veterinary oversight of the use of antibiotics in apiculture.
- The definition of prescription and veterinary feed directive (VFD) use in apiculture.
- The description of approved veterinary antibiotic formulations for use in honey bees in the United States and Canada.
- A practical summary provision of the indications, dosage, cautions, and applications of approved veterinary antibiotics in honey bees.
- Descriptions of medications that do not require veterinary prescriptions or VFDs but are commonly used by beekeepers to treat a variety of medical conditions in honey bees.

INTRODUCTION AND HISTORY

In January 2017, the US Food and Drug Administration (FDA) mandate requiring veterinary oversight of medically important antibiotics came into effect. This mandate included honey bees (*Apis mellifera L.*) as agricultural animals.[1,2] A similar mandate occurred in Canada in December of 2018. There are 3 antibiotics labeled for honey bees requiring veterinary oversight in both the United States and Canada.[3,4]

Antibiotics can be issued by veterinarians to beekeepers for their honey bees if a valid veterinary-client-patient relationship (VCPR) exists. Requirements for VCPR can vary state to state and province to province. In the United States, the federal definition of VCPR minimally applies in the States (**Box 1**). In some situations and locations, telemedicine may be used to serve beekeepers; however, in the United States, VCPRs are *initially* established with on-site visits.[5]

Before the FDA mandate, apiarists/inspectors could recommend and administer antibiotics to affected hives. Since the mandate, they are no longer legally allowed to do

Grove City College, 100 Campus Drive, Grove City, PA 16127, USA
E-mail address: tsfarone@gcc.edu

Vet Clin Food Anim 37 (2021) 451–465
https://doi.org/10.1016/j.cvfa.2021.06.009
0749-0720/21/© 2021 Elsevier Inc. All rights reserved.
vetfood.theclinics.com

Box 1
The federal definition of a valid veterinary-client-patient relationship

"A veterinarian has assumed the responsibility for making medical judgments regarding the health of (an) animal(s) and the need for medical treatment, and the client (the owner of the animal or animals or other caretaker) has agreed to follow the instructions of the veterinarian;

There is sufficient knowledge of the animal(s) by the veterinarian to initiate at least a general or preliminary diagnosis of the medical condition of the animal(s); and

The practicing veterinarian is readily available for follow up in case of adverse reactions or failure of the regimen of therapy. Such a relationship can exist only when the veterinarian has recently seen and is personally acquainted with the keeping and care of the animal(s) by virtue of examination of the animal(s), and/or by medically appropriate and timely visits to the premises where the animal(s) are kept."

Data from Electronic Code of Federal Regulations. Ecfr.gov. 2020. Available at: https://www. ecfr.gov/cgi-bin/text-idx?SID=99550a83c97103df1503d4e34b99b26b Accessed December 09.

---

so. Veterinarians interested in seeing honey bees should become familiar with their local state bee inspector in order to work as a team. The Apiary Inspectors of America (https://apiaryinspectors.org/) is a nonprofit organization that provides valuable resources for regulations, laws, and programs at the national and state level.[6]

DISCUSSION

Antibiotics can be issued via a prescription or veterinary feed directive (VFD). VFDs are required for antibiotics approved and formulated for use in or on feed products. Prescriptions are used for antibiotic formulations not for use in feed. Water additives are considered prescription products but may be used as dry dustings in honey bees.[7] Because honey bees are given antibiotics in the form of dustings of sugar and/or sugar syrup, distinction between VFDs and prescriptions can seem somewhat blurred. The best advice is for the practitioner to become familiar with the formulations and their VFD or prescription designations.

Labels and indications for antibiotic use must be followed. It is the law but also good practice in providing the safest course of treatment of honey bees, preventing drug resistance, and preventing residues in honey bee products.[1,8,9] When writing a VFD be sure to copy instructions exactly as on the label of the medication. Regulations require VFDs to expire within 6 months from the date of issue. Once signed, veterinarians should keep a record of the VFD for 2 years and provide copies to the client and distributor. Regarding prescriptions, it is highly recommended that labels are followed; however, some allowance for extralabel use may be permitted, because honey bees are considered a minor species.[8,10,11] Helpful and specific information on licensed drug distributors and drug label instructions (Blue Bird Labels) can be found using the following links:

Detailed Blue Bird labels https://animaldrugsatfda.fda.gov/adafda/views/#/home/previewsearch/008-804.
Licensed distributors by State https://animaldrugsatfda.fda.gov/adafda/app/search/public/vfdPdfByStateName/vfdByStateName.

VFD drugs are type A medicated articles and are not intended for administration to honey bees before proper mixing with a feed. Type A medicated articles, intended to be mixed into feed to produce type B (which requires further dilution before administration) or type C medicated feed, are available. Attention should be paid to sourcing and purchasing medicated feeds, as some honey bee suppliers may be selling type A medicated articles. These products are intended to be sold to a licensed distributor and not directly to a consumer.

Type C medicated feeds are ready to be sold to the client and administered to the intended population. Several type C medicated feeds are available from bee supply distributors in conveniently sized packaging for small scale beekeepers and larger quantities available for commercial operations. Be sure to choose medicated products that are practical for use in your client's situation. More information about type A and C medicated feeds can be found in the USDA veterinary accreditation module #29 at https://nvap.aphis.usda.gov/VFD/index.htm.

There are many proprietors of honey bee products within the United States and Canada, many of which also sell and distribute antibiotics for honey bees. These companies stock, have access to, and can sell antibiotics directly to beekeepers with a prescription or VFD. Approved indications of these drugs can be used for prevention, control, and/or treatment of disease; this is of primary importance in the management of foulbrood in migratory and/or commercial operations.[1,3,4,8]

The 3 approved drugs for use in honey bees are oxytetracycline, tylosin, and lincomycin. They are available in 11 different approved veterinary preparations. Directions, dosage, applications, and duration for each antibiotic preparation are contained in **Table 1**.[12]

The following points are summarized from **Table 1**:

- Only one drug, oxytetracycline, is approved for the treatment of *Melissococcus plutonius*, the etiologic agent of European foulbrood (EFB), by either a VFD or prescription.
- For *Paenibacillus larvae*, the etiologic agent of American foulbrood (AFB), oxytetracycline is approved in both VFD and prescription forms.
- Tylosin and lincomycin can be used for AFB by prescription only.
- Some states' Departments of Agriculture or Provinces may require beekeepers to burn AFB diagnosed hives with no option of antibiotic treatment.[12]

Keep in mind that indications and administrative instructions for antibiotic uses in honey bees are based on preventative treatments for AFB/EFB in the spring and fall. Treatment with tylosin should only be completed in the fall, as there is the potential for drug residues in summer honey if administered in the spring.[1,7] As veterinarians, we may also be called on to treat outbreaks at any time of the year and must make the client aware of withdraw time implications. Antibiotics cannot be used when honey supers are on and must be withdrawn 4 to 6 weeks *before* honey supers are added. Withdrawal time starts with the completion of the last treatment.[1,9,12] Honey produced during treatment times should not be used for human consumption, and this requires careful management planning and record keeping.[1,7] Veterinarians can play an important role in educating beekeepers on the importance of good antibiotic stewardship to reduce antibiotic resistance and antibiotic residues for the best health of honey bees and honey bee product consumers.

CLINICAL RELEVANCE OF TREATMENT

Antibiotics do not kill AFB spores; they only affect the vegetative infection in the larvae, potentially suppressing clinical disease. If antibiotic treatment is discontinued in a spore-laden hive, clinical AFB may develop. This is why many beekeepers are reluctant to stop "preventative" treatment on their colonies. However, overuse or misuse of oxytetracycline has also led to antibiotic resistance for *P larvae*, further contributing to

Table 1
Antibiotics approved for use in honey bees

Application#	Trade Name	Active Ingredient	Disease	Dosage/Administration	Rx/VFD	WDT
008-804	TM-10, TM-50, TM-50D, TM-100, TM-100D, TM-100SS	Oxytetracycline hydrochloride	AFB/EFB	Use 200 mg Terramycin/colony. Consult with label for application directions	VFD	42 d before main nectar flow
095-143	TERRAMYCIN 10, TERRAMYCIN 30, TERRAMYCIN 50, TERRAMYCIN 100, TERRAMYCIN 200, TERRAMYCIN 200 Granular, TERRAMYCIN 100MR, OXTC-100MR, OXTC-200, OXTC-50, OXTC-100-S	Oxytetracycline hydrochloride	AFB/EFB	Use 200 mg Terramycin/colony. Consult with label for application directions	VFD	42 d before main nectar flow
138-938	Pennox 50, Pennox 100MR, Pennox 100 Hi-flo, Pennox 200 Hi-flo	Oxytetracycline hydrochloride	AFB/EFB	Use 200 mg Pennox/colony. Consult with label for application directions	VFD	42 d before main nectar flow
200-146	Tetroxy 25, Oxytetracycline HCl Soluble Powder	Oxytetracycline hydrochloride	AFB/EFB	Use 200 mg of Tetroxy/colony. Administer via either a 1:1 sugar syrup or dust the top bar of the brood frames with a powdered sugar mixture. Tetroxy should be administered in 3 applications of sugar syrup or 3 dustings at 4- to 5-d intervals. Do not apply dusting to uncapped brood as it can cause death.	Rx	42 d before main nectar flow
200-247	Tetroxy 343	Oxytetracycline hydrochloride	AFB/EFB	Use 200 mg of Tetroxy/colony. Administer via either a 1:1 sugar syrup or dust the top bar of the brood frames with a powdered sugar mixture. Tetroxy should be administered in 3 applications of sugar syrup or 3 dustings at 4- to 5-d intervals. Do not apply dusting to uncapped brood as it can cause death.	Rx	42 d before main nectar flow

008-622	TERRAMYCIN-343, TERRAMYCIN, TERRAMYCIN Soluble Powder Concentrate	Oxytetracycline hydrochloride	AFB	Use 200 mg Terramycin/colony. Administer via either a 1:1 sugar syrup or dust the top bar of the brood frames with a powdered sugar mixture. Terramycin should be administered in 3 applications of sugar syrup or 3 dustings at 4- to 5-d intervals. Do not apply dusting to uncapped brood as it can cause death.	Rx	42 d before main nectar flow
200-026	Pennox 343	Oxytetracycline hydrochloride	AFB	Use 200 mg of Pennox/colony. Administer via either a 1:1 sugar syrup or dust the top bar of the brood frames with a powdered sugar mixture. Pennox should be administered in 3 applications of sugar syrup or 3 dustings at 4- to 5-d intervals. Do not apply dusting to uncapped brood as it can cause death.	Rx	42 d before main nectar flow
013-076	Tylan Soluble	Tylosin tartrate	AFB	Use 200 mg/colony of Tylan mixed with 20g powdered sugar. Colonies should receive 3 treatments administered as a dust over the top bar of the brood frames once a week for 3 wk. Do not apply mixture to uncapped brood as it can cause death.	Rx	28 d before main nectar flow
200-455	BiloVet, Tylosin Tartrate Soluble Powder	Tylosin tartrate	AFB	Mix 200 mg tylosin in 20 g of powdered sugar. Apply dust to the top bar of the brood frame. BiloVet should be administered once weekly for 3 wk. Do not apply dusting to uncapped brood as it can cause death.	Rx	28 d before main nectar flow

(continued on next page)

Table 1
(continued)

Application#	Trade Name	Active Ingredient	Disease	Dosage/Administration	Rx/VFD	WDT
200-473	Tylovet Soluble	Tylosin tartrate	AFB	Mix 200 mg Tylovet/colony in 20 g powdered sugar. Use immediately. Apply dust to the top bar of the brood frame. Tylovet should be administered once weekly for 3 wk. Do not apply dusting to uncapped brood as it can cause death.	Rx	28 d before main nectar flow
111-636	LINCOMIX Soluble Powder	Lincomycin hydrochloride	AFB	Mix 100 mg of lincomycin with 20 g of powdered sugar. Dust over the top bar of the brood frames once a week for 3 wk. Do not apply mixture to uncapped brood as it can cause death.	Rx	28 d before main nectar flow

Important note: use all antibiotic mixtures immediately.

Data from Animal Drugs @ FDA. Animaldrugsatfda.fda.gov. 2020. Available at: https://animaldrugsatfda.fda.gov/adafda/views/#home/searchResult. Accessed December 9, 2020. & Honey Bees: Approved FDA Drugs. Farad.org. 2020. Available at: http://www.farad.org/vetgram/honeybees.asp. Accessed December 11th, 2020.

the ineffectiveness of using antibiotic treatments in honey bees.[13,14] Veterinarians play key roles in directing and advocating for good antibiotic stewardship with honey bees and beekeepers.

The drugs, pesticides, and other chemicals that are used to treat honey bee diseases can leave residues and contaminate bee products, such as honey and wax. Similar to antibiotics, many drugs, such as certain miticides, cannot be used when honey supers are on or must be withdrawn 4 to 6 weeks before honey supers are added. Veterinarians can work with beekeepers to improve the management, planning, and record keeping of drug administration to achieve proper use, maximal effectiveness, and safety of the medications used in honey bees.

NATURE OF THE PROBLEM, CONTROVERSIES, AND APPROACH

If AFB is suspected in the field, immediate action should ensue. The state/provincial apiarist should be contacted and specific state or provincial and federal laws should be followed for disease management. State/provincial apiarists, the beekeepers, and veterinarians should all work together to be sure proper protocols are followed and samples are also sent off for laboratory confirmation of AFB.

Be aware that the use of antibiotics in honey bees has been associated with a variety of side effects, including death of brood, decreased lifespan, and dysbiosis through disruption of normal gut flora.[14,15] Drugs are only one tool in our toolbox for fighting disease. Integrated pest management is a practice commonly used by beekeepers and veterinarians. Using multiple modalities to manage or treat pests or disease may help to attain positive clinical outcomes and reduce the reliance on any one facet of the protocol. Engaging in best management practices of biosecurity, requeening, proper nutrition, and sometimes benign neglect may be complimentary when developing a treatment plan.[15–17]

OTHER PRODUCTS COMMONLY USED IN THE TREATMENT OF HONEY BEES

Because veterinarians should be aware of all aspects of their patient's health, it is highly recommended that the practitioner develop a comprehensive understanding of honey bee maladies and the medications and pesticides commonly used by beekeepers to address these health issues. Keen awareness of all potential diseases and chemical use certainly contributes to the overall assessment of the patient, differential diagnoses, and successful treatment.

Tables 2–4 have been provided to summarize nonantimicrobial drugs and pesticides commonly used to treat honey bees that are not under the purview of veterinarians. Although veterinary oversight is not required for beekeepers to obtain over-the-counter drugs and pesticides in the United States and Canada, veterinarians should be equipped to aid beekeepers in making best practice treatment choices regarding these chemicals.

FOR VARROA MITES, *VARROA DESTRUCTOR*, VARROOSIS

Varroosis is the single largest disease threat and the major contributor to colony loss in the world.[1,5,16–19] It is typical and most effective for beekeepers to use different chemicals at multiple times over the course of a beekeeping season to keep Varroa mites under control.[18,19] Various products have differing ideal and proper use times during the beekeeping season. Temperature, brood cycle, and if honey supers are in use are all considerations for treatment selection and timing.[18,19] Rotation of chemical treatment is recommended to help reduce the development of drug resistance.[1,18,19]

Table 2
Common products used in the treatment of varroosis

Registration #	Trade Name	Active Ingredient	Application Method	Treat While Honey Supers On?	Dosage/Administration
2724-406	Zoecon rf-318 Apistan strip, Apistan Anti-Varroa Mite Strips	Fluvalinate (10.25%)	Use 1 strip for every 5 frames of bees. Leave on for 6 wk	No	Use at the end of the season. Rotate with other treatments to reduce resistance
73291-1	Api Life VAR	Thymol (74.09%), oil of eucalyptus (16%), Menthol (3.73%)	Use 3 wafers per colony. Place wafers in the corners of the brood box. Use once a week for 3 consecutive wk, replacing with new wafers each time	No	Use in temperatures between 65° and 95° F. If bees try to remove wafers, block wafers with wire mesh. Best if rotated with other treatments
75710-2	Mite-Away Quick Strips	Formic acid (46.7%)	Place 2 strips over the top of the brood frames. Remove after 7 d	Yes	Hive must have bee clusters that cover at least 6 brood frames. Use in temperatures between 50° and 84° F
75710-3	Formic Pro	Formic acid (42.25%)	Lay strips across the top of the brood frames. Can use 2 strips for 14 d or 1 strip for 10 d followed by a second strip for an additional 10 d	Yes	Use in temperatures between 50° and 84° F
79671-1	Apiguard	Thymol (25%)	Place tray on top of the brood frame. Leave in the hive for 10–14 d then replace with a second tray. Leave the second tray on for 2–4 wk	No	Use in temperatures between 60° and 100° F. Best if rotated with other treatments
83623-2	Hopguard 2	Hop beta acids resin (16%)	Hang 2 strips per 10 frames of bees. Hang only in the brood frames. Leave on for 5–7 d	Yes	Use when the daytime temperature is higher than 50°F. Rotate with other treatments

87243-1	Apivar	Amitraz (3.33%)	Hang 2 strips per brood chamber. Remove after 42 d	No	Use in temperatures between 59° and 100° F
91266-1	Oxalic Acid Dihydrate	Oxalic acid (100%)	Perform one treatment once a week for 3 consecutive weeks via drip or with a vaporizer	No	Drip form cannot be used in temperatures less than 55° F. Does not kill mites under cappings. Best used during late fall or early spring
11556-138	Checkmite + Bee Hive Pest Control Strip	Coumaphos (10%)	Use 1 strip for every 5 frames of bees. Remove strips after 42–45 d	No	Wait 2 wk after treatment ends to add honey supers. For best use, use at the end of the season when brood levels are low

Data from EPA-registered Pesticide Products Approved for Use Against Varroa Mites in Bee Hives. Epa.gov. 2018. Available at: https://www.epa.gov/pollinator-protection/epa-registered-pesticide-products-approved-use-against-varroa-mites-bee-hives. Accessed December 10th, 2020. and Tools for Varroa Management: A Guide to Effective Varroa Sampling & Control. HoneyBeeHelathCoalition.org. 2018. Available at: https://honeybeehealthcoalition.org/wp-content/uploads/2018/06/HBHC-Guide_Varroa_Interactive_7thEdition_June2018.pdf. Accessed December 10th, 2020.

Table 3
Common products in the treatment of hive beetles

Registration #	Trade Name	Active Ingredient	Application Method	Dosage/Administration
—	Beetle Baffle	—	With the angled edges facing down, place the metal side rails along the top of the wood space. Do the same with the end rails making sure to overlap with the side rails. Staple or nail it together	Make sure to fasten the rails to the wood with 3 fasteners on each rail
—	Beetle Blaster	—	Place trap between 2 frames in the hive and fill with beetle trap oil. Throw away once full	Can be used at any time during the season
—	Beetle Towel	—	Cut each towel sheet into 3 equal strips. Place 6 of these strips in a hive at a time	The Bees will chew on the towel and the beetles will get caught in the towel. Remember to remove strips periodically
11556-138	Checkmite+	Coumaphos (10%)	Use 1 strip for every 5 frames of bees. Remove strips after 42–45 d	Wait 2 wk after treatment ends to add honey supers. For best use, use at the end of the season when brood levels are low. Do not use while honey supers are on
39039-8	GardStar	Permethrin	Check label for dilution instructions. Use on the soil surrounding the hives. Reapply as needed every 30–90 d	Permethrin is toxic to bees. Avoid sprinkling on surfaces the bees come into contact with. Apply with a sprinkler can in the late evening

Data from Hive Beetle. Mannlakeltd.com. 2020. Available at: https://www.mannlakeltd.com/shop-all-categories/hive-colony-maintenance/medications-treatments-herbicides/hive-beetle. Accessed December 12th, 2020. & Small Hive Beetle. agdev.anr.udel.edu. 2015. Available at:https://agdev.anr.udel.edu/maarec/wp- content/uploads/2010/05/SMALL_HIVE_BEETLE_FACT_SHEET_1-29.pdf. Accessed December 11th, 2020.

Table 4
Common products used in the treatment of wax moths

Registration #	Trade Name	Active Ingredient	Application Method	Dosage/ Administration
61671-2	Para-Moth	Para-dichlorobenzene	Place crystals on a paper plate and place on the top bars of the topmost super and cover with a tarp	Supers should be stacked in groups of 5–9 depending on the depth. Allow equipment to air out for several days before use
—	Certan	Bacillus thuringiensis	Use after honey extraction. Spray a thin layer of diluted Certan on both sides of the frame. Allow to dry before storing	Dilute to 5% before use and use the same day
—	Freezing method	–	Place frames in a freezer until they reach temperatures of 20°F for 4.5 h, 10°F for 3 h, or 5°F for 2 h	Kills all life stages of wax moths. Store freeze treated frames in a cool, bright, well-ventilated place if not using immediately

Data from Wax Moths. Mannlakeltd.com. 2020. Available at: https://www.mannlakeltd.com/shop-all-categories/hive-colony-maintenance/medications-treatments-herbicides/wax-moths. Accessed December 11th, 2020 & Hood, M. Wax Moth IPM. Clemson.edu. 2010. Available at: https://www.clemson.edu/extension/beekeepers/fact-sheets-publications/wax-moth-ipm-publication.html. Accessed December 11th, 2020.

Table 2 provides the names of formulations of products, indications, application, dosage, and duration of use for products used to control Varroa mites.[19,20]

Some varroa control products, such as fluvalinate and coumaphos, have widely reported resistance issues.[4] Some beekeepers may use a product called Taktic, which contains amitraz, to control varroa mites. This product is considered low cost but is not an approved product for use in honey bees.[20]

FOR SMALL HIVE BEETLE, *AETHINA TUMIDA*, INFESTATIONS

Small hive beetles are considered ubiquitous across much of the United States and often viewed as a nuisance pest that can be managed but unlikely eliminated. Preventative management strategies (biosecurity) and traps can help control small hive beetles without the use of chemicals.[21,22] When chemical control is used, consideration should be given to bee toxicity and the risk of residues in hive products.[21,22] Pollen patties infested with small hive beetle should be removed and destroyed.[21,22] **Table 3** provides the names of formulations of products, indications, application, dosage, and duration of use of products used to control hive beetles.[21]

NOSEMOSIS: NOSEMA APIS, NOSEMA CERANAE

Maintaining strong colonies and providing proper ventilation, sanitation, and good nutrition are the mainstays in prevention and treatment of Nosemosis in honey bees.[17,23] The antibiotic, fumagillin (Fumidil B), is available for treatment of Nosema.[3,4] Even though fumagillin is an antibiotic, it does not require a VFD or a prescription from a veterinarian because it is not classified as a medically important antibiotic (for humans).[1,10] Fumagillin can be used to treat colonies in the fall and/or early spring. Various dosing protocols exist; consult the label for detailed administration[24].

Fumagillin is not effective in killing Nosema spores; therefore, it may not be effective in treating heavily infected colonies.[17,23] Some research shows that fumagillin is not effective and may worsen infection in the treatment of *N ceranae*, which may be becoming the more common species of Nosema infections seen in honey bees.[17,23,25] Fumagillin should not be used when supers are on or within the specified withdrawal period before a honey flow due to risk of drug residues.[17,23]

TRACHEAL MITES, *ACARAPIS WOODI*

Tracheal mite infestations have fallen out of focus after the emergence of Varroa mites. Fortunately, many of the products used to control Varroa mites also control tracheal mites.[24,26,27] Currently, a single product on the market, Mite-A-Thol (Menthol) is indicated for the treatment of tracheal mites.[26,27] Packets are placed on top bars of the top hive box for 28 days. Treatment should be done in temperatures between 60 and 80° Fahrenheit. Be sure to follow all labeled instructions.[26,27] Mite-A-Thol should not be used if honey supers are on or 4 weeks before nectar flow.[26,27]

GREATER WAX MOTH, *GALLERIA MELLONELLA*, AND LESSER WAX MOTH, *ACHROIA GRISELLA*

No chemical treatments are approved for use in live colonies.[28–30] In small operations, hygienic frame care with proper storage, cleaning, exposure to ultraviolet light and freezing is the best and chemical free way of controlling this opportunistic parasite.[28–30] **Table 4** provides the names of formulations of products, indications, application, dosage, and duration of use for products used to control wax moths.[28]

CANADIAN PRODUCTS

Many of the medicated products approved and available for use in the United States are similar or the same in Canada. There are, however, a few differences. Oxytetracycline, tylosin, and lincomycin are available only by veterinary prescription, as there are no VFD drugs or feed designations in Canada, and some provinces do not require site visits to establish VCPRs. Similar to the United States, hive products for treatment of Varroa, Nosema, and other pests are also available but do not require veterinary oversight.[31,32]

FUTURE DIRECTIONS

Honey bee veterinary medicine is a developing field in the United States and Canada since the legislative changes of 2017 and 2018, respectively, requiring veterinary oversight of medically important antibiotics in apiculture. At the time of this writing, many US and Canadian veterinary schools are beginning to add honey bee medicine into their curriculum, and continuing education is largely available for veterinarians. Professional groups of veterinarians willing to see bees have been formed.[33] As more veterinarians become equipped in honey bee medicine, they will serve as a valuable ally to the apicultural industry, responsible antibiotic stewardship, and One Health priorities.

CLINICS CARE POINTS, CAUTIONS, AND TIPS

- To simplify matters, find and become familiar with the use of a VFD and/or prescription formulation for each antibiotic that you can easily obtain from a supplier.
- Antibiotics may be available in large bag sizes, some greater than 50 lbs per bag. However, the dosage to treat a single colony only requires a small amount. Be aware large package sizes could lead to excessive amounts of drug distributed and possible stockpiling.[1,7,9]
- If using soluble powder formulations in syrup, dissolve the antibiotic powder in a small amount of water before adding to the syrup.[12]
- Extender patties are available for delivery of oxytetracycline. Extender patties are premade articles impregnated with a drug that is placed in a hive to deliver medications over time. This method of delivery is not recommended for antibiotics due to the persistence of drug residues and potential development of antibiotic resistance.[1]

ACKNOWLEDGMENTS

Ms Katerina Bailey (senior biology research student and GCC apiary manager) for her assistance with the chapter's literary review and table creation.

DISCLOSURE

The author has nothing to disclose.

REFERENCES

1. Honey bees: a guide for veterinarians. AVMA.org. 2017. Available at: https://www.avma.org/sites/default/files/resources/honeybees-veterinary-medicine-guide-for-veterinarians.pdf. Accessed December 10, 2020.
2. Honey bees 101 for veterinarians. AVMA.org. Available at: https://www.avma.org/honey-bees-101-veterinarians. Accessed December 10, 2020.
3. Registered medications and pesticides for honey bee health in the United States. Honeybeehealthcoalition.org. Available at: https://honeybeehealthcoalition.org/wp-content/uploads/2020/10/HBHC_Approved_Medications_US_092320.pdf. Accessed December 11, 2020.
4. Registered medications and pesticides for honey bee health in Canada. Honeybeehealthcoalition.org. Available at: https://honeybeehealthcoalition.org/wp-content/uploads/2020/10/HBHC_Approved_Medications_Canada_092320.pdf. Accessed December 11, 2020.
5. Module 30: the role of veterinarians in honey bee health. Nvap.aphis.usda.gov. 2020. Available at: https://nvap.aphis.usda.gov/BEE/bee0001.php. Accessed December 11, 2020.
6. Apiary inspectors of America. Apiaryinspectors.org. Available at: https://apiaryinspectors.org/. Accessed December 10, 2020.
7. Using medically important antimicrobials in bees. Fda.gov. Available at: https://www.fda.gov/animal-veterinary/development-approval-process/using-medically-important-antimicrobials-bees-questions-and-answers. Accessed December 11, 2020.

8. Module 29: veterinary feed directive. Nvap.aphis.usda.gov. 2020. Available at: https://nvap.aphis.usda.gov/VFD/index.htm. Accessed December 11, 2020.

9. Module 23: use of antibiotics in animals. Nvap.aphis.usda.gov. 2020. Available at: https://nvap.aphis.usda.gov/ABX/index.htm. Accessed December 11, 2020.

10. Veterinary Feed Directive (VFD). FDA.gov. 2020. Available at: https://www.fda.gov/animal-veterinary/development-approval-process/veterinary-feed-directive-vfd. Accessed December 10, 2020.

11. Extralabel drug use in animals. Ecfr.gov. 2020. Available at: https://www.ecfr.gov/cgi-bin/textidx?SID=ed376126689421877963a701086a316e&mc=true&node=pt21.6.530&rgn=div5. Accessed December 10, 2020.

12. Honey bees: approved FDA drugs. Farad.org. 2020. Available at: http://www.farad.org/vetgram/honeybees.asp. Accessed December 11, 2020.

13. Feeding sugar to honey bees August 2014, Primefact 1343 first edition Doug Somerville, Technical Specialist Honey Bees Intensive Livestock, Goulburn, Feeding sugar to honey bees. Available at: nsw.gov.au. Accessed December 16, 2020.

14. Tian B, Fadhil NH, Powell JE, et al. Long-term exposure to antibiotics has caused accumulation of resistance determinants in the gut microbiota of honeybees. mBio 2012;3(6):e00377.

15. Raymann K, Shaffer Z, Moran NA. Antibiotic exposure perturbs the gut microbiota and elevates mortality in honeybees. PLOS Biol 2017;15(3):e2001861.

16. Sallmann B, Snyder R. In: Rennich K, Caron DM, Lee K, et al, editors. Diagnosis and treatment of common honey bee diseases. Bee Informed Partnership, Inc; 2014.

17. Vidal-Naquet N. Honeybee veterinary medicine: Apis mellifera. Sheffield, UK: 5m Publishing; 2015.

18. Tools for varroa management: a guide to effective varroa sampling & control. HoneyBeeHelathCoalition.org. Available at: https://honeybeehealthcoalition.org/wp-content/uploads/2018/06/HBHC-Guide_Varroa_Interactive_7thEdition_June2018.pdf. Accessed December 10, 2020.

19. Ambrose J, Tarpy D, Summers J, et al. Managing varroa mites in honey bee colonies. Extension.Iastate.edu. 2017. Available at: https://www.extension.iastate.edu/smallfarms/managing-varroa-mites-honey-bee-colonies. Accessed December 11, 2020.

20. EPA-registered pesticide products approved for use against varroa mites in bee hives. Epa.gov. 2018. Available at: https://www.epa.gov/pollinator-protection/epa-registered-pesticide-products-approved-use-against-varroa-mites-bee-hives. Accessed December 10, 2020.

21. Small hive beetle. agdev.anr.udel.edu. 2015. Available at: https://agdev.anr.udel.edu/maarec/wp-content/uploads/2010/05/SMALL_HIVE_BEETLE_FACT_SHEET_1-29.pdf. Accessed December 11, 2020.

22. Zawislak J. Managing small hive beetles. Bee-health.extension.org. 2019. Available at: https://bee-health.extension.org/managing-small-hive-beetles/. Accessed December 11, 2020.

23. Huang Z. How is Nosema disease treated? Bee-health.extension.org 2019. Available at: https://bee-health.extension.org/how-is-nosema-disease-treated/. Accessed December 11, 2020.

24. Huang W, Solter LF, Yau PM, et al. Nosema ceranae escapes fumagillin control in honey bees. PLoS Pathog 2013;9(3):e1003185.

25. Hood W. Honey bee tracheal mite. Clemson.edu 2000. Available at: https://www. clemson.edu/extension/beekeepers/fact-sheets-publications/tracheal-mite-honey-bee.html. Accessed December 11, 2020.
26. Moore P, Wilson ME, Skinner JA, et al. Honey bee tracheal mites: gone? But not for good. Bee-health.extension.org 2019. Available at: https://bee-health. extension.org/honey-bee-tracheal-mites-gone-but-not-for-good/.   Accessed December 11, 2020.
27. Tracheal Mite. Ars.usda.gov. 2016. Available at: https://www.ars.usda.gov/ northeast-area/beltsville-md-barc/beltsville-agricultural-research-center/bee-research-laboratory/docs/tracheal-mite/. Accessed December 11, 2020.
28. Hood M. Wax Moth IPM. Clemson.edu. 2010. Available at: https://www.clemson. edu/extension/beekeepers/fact-sheets-publications/wax-moth-ipm-publication. html. Accessed December 11, 2020.
29. Wax moth a beekeeping pest. Agriculture.vic.gov.au. Available at: https:// agriculture.vic.gov.au/biosecurity/pest-insects-and-mites/priority-pest-insects-and-mites/wax-moth-a-beekeeping-pest. Accessed December 11, 2020.
30. Cameron J, Ellis J. Wax Moth Control. Edis.ifas.ufl.edu. 2018. Available at: https:// edis.ifas.ufl.edu/aa141. Accessed December 11, 2020.
31. Registered chemicals and drugs in beekeeping. Gov.Bc.Ca. Available at: https:// www2.gov.bc.ca/assets/gov/farming-natural-resources-and-industry/agriculture-and-seafood/animal-and-crops/animal-production/bee-assets/api_fs004.pdf? bcgovtm=CSMLS. Accessed December 10, 2020.
32. Recommendations for administering antibiotics and Acaricides to honey. Lafre-nière, Rhéal, and ostermann, David, Manitoba agriculture. Available at: https:// www.gov.mb.ca/agriculture/crops/crop-management/pubs/administering-antibiotics-and-acaricides-to-honey-bees.pdf. Accessed February 25, 2021.
33. The honey bee veterinary consortium. Available at: https://www.hbvc.org/. Ac-cessed December 17, 2020.

Working with State and Provincial Apiary Programs to Manage Honey Bee (*Apis mellifera*) Health

Kim Skyrm, PhD[a,*], Natasha Garcia-Andersen, BS[b],
Mary Reed, BS[c], Tammy Horn Potter, PhD[d], Brooke Decker, MS[e],
Jennifer Lund, MS[f]

KEYWORDS

- Honey bee • Apiarist • Apiary inspector • Apiary program

KEY POINTS

- Beekeeping is an important agricultural business that provides pollination services for many crops and wildflowers, honey, hive products, and bees.
- Most states, territories, and provinces have laws and regulations pertaining to honey bee health and beekeeping.
- Apiary inspectors and apiary programs are primarily responsible for enforcing the laws and regulations of certain honey bee pests and diseases. Apiarists also often serve as educators, researchers, state fair superintendents, and coordinators for other-bee related activities, such as Managed Pollinator Protection Plans.
- As a result of the Food and Drug Administration Veterinary Feed Directive (VFD), which went into effect in 2017, beekeepers now are required to obtain a VFD or veterinarian's prescription to purchase antibiotics used to manage American foulbrood or European foulbrood. Apiary inspectors are eager to collaborate with veterinarians in facilitating and fulfilling legal requirements of the VFD (or prescription).
- Communication between apiarists and veterinarians is key to managing healthy honey bee colonies and controlling disease outbreaks when they occur.

[a] Massachusetts Department of Agricultural Resources, 138 Memorial Avenue, Suite 42, West Springfield, MA 01089, USA; [b] Department of Energy and Environment, 1200 First Street Northeast, 5th Floor, Washington, DC 20002, USA; [c] Texas Apiary Inspection Service, 2475 Texas A&M University, College Station, TX 77843-2475, USA; [d] Kentucky Department of Agriculture, 109 Corporate Drive, Frankfort, KY 40601, USA; [e] Vermont Agency of Agriculture, Food and Markets, 116 State Street, Montpelier, VT 05620-2901, USA; [f] Maine Department of Agriculture, Conservation and Forestry, 18 Elkins Lane, Augusta, ME 04330, USA
* Corresponding author.
E-mail address: kim.skyrm@mass.gov

Vet Clin Food Anim 37 (2021) 467–478
https://doi.org/10.1016/j.cvfa.2021.06.003
0749-0720/21/Published by Elsevier Inc.

BACKGROUND

Commercial beekeeping is an important and viable business throughout North America. In the United States, products and services the beekeeping industry provides contribute significantly to the GDP and are estimated to be valued at $4.74 billion.[1] Over the past several years, there has been an increasing demand for Western honey bees (*Apis mellifera*), for both pollination of crops and honey production. The beekeeping industry is facing many challenges, however, the most significant of which is honey bee health. The management of honey bee health issues and the interstate movement of hives throughout North America is regulated by officials known as apiarists, apiculturists, or apiary inspectors (hereafter referred to collectively as *apiary inspectors*). Most apiary or bee inspection programs (hereafter referred to collectively as *apiary programs*) are affiliated with either government or university programs. The first apiary program and bee laws in North America were established in California in 1877 in response to a highly contagious and deadly bacterial disease, known as American foulbrood (AFB), caused by the etiologic agent *Paenibacillus larvae*, which was responsible for colony deaths and corresponding catastrophic economic losses for beekeepers (**Fig. 1**).[2] AFB had been identified as a problem prior to 1877, but as the economic viability of beekeeping grew, state lawmakers began to establish enforceable measures to help mitigate its spread. Over the following decades, several other states, provinces, and territories followed California's lead in developing apiary programs.

During the 1960s to 1990s, the economic viability of commercial scale beekeeping and interstate transport of hives in North America increased and backyard or hobby beekeeping saw a surge in interest. There was a corresponding sharp increase in

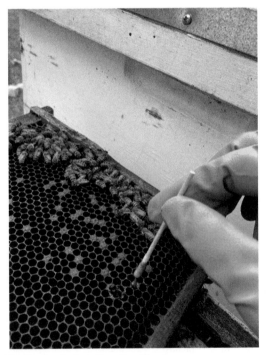

Fig. 1. AFB, caused by the bacterium *Paenibacillus larvae*.

cases of AFB and another unrelated bacterial disease, European foulbrood (EFB), caused by the bacterium *Melissococcus plutonius*, across North America (**Fig. 2**). The primary tool used by beekeepers for both AFB and EFB management has been the antibiotic oxytetracycline.[3] Although an effective management tool for EFB, a non–spore-forming bacteria, oxytetracycline does not cure infection with AFB, which is a spore-forming bacteria. Oxytetracycline suppresses AFB symptoms and requires regular, twice-yearly applications. At times, AFB was so widespread that if a beekeeper did not manage the disease, the hive likely would die from infection, and AFB potentially would spread to neighboring hives. This practice was neither sustainable nor good animal husbandry. As a result, the beekeeping industry petitioned local governments to start or revamp apiary programs. Many states, provinces, and territories responded, which led to the modern iteration of most apiary programs throughout North America. Since the late 1980s, detections of AFB have decreased throughout North America as apiary programs implemented AFB mitigation plans in their respective states, provinces, and territories.

In the 2010s, the Food and Drug Administration (FDA) became concerned with medically important antibiotic use in livestock management. In 2015, the FDA amended the Animal Drug Availability Act of 1996 to include revisions to the Veterinary Feed Directive (VFD) section of the regulation.[4] Similar changes were made in 2017 for Canada's Food and Drug Act Amendments.[5] The revisions limited the use of antibiotics in or on animal feed and required the supervision of a licensed veterinarian for the administration of medically important antibiotics to livestock, including honey bees.

As a result of the VFD, beekeepers and veterinarians have relied on apiary inspectors for clarification of the federal directive. Some states or provinces have a single

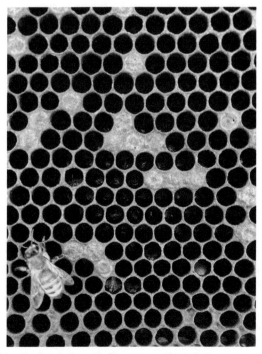

Fig. 2. EFB, caused by the bacterium *Melissococcus plutonius*.

apiarist or apiary inspector, whereas others have a chief apiary inspector and several regional apiary inspectors forming a collective apiary program. The chief apiary inspector coordinates the apiary program and oversees seasonal, full-time, or part-time positions based on need and funding. For states, provinces, and territories that do not have apiary programs, government or university-affiliated animal or plant health inspectors perform this role, as needed.

Similar to that of a veterinarian, the primary role of an apiary inspector is to ensure the health and well-being of animals, specifically honey bees. Even though apiary inspectors typically do not receive formal veterinary medicine education and are not considered medical professionals, they often are highly trained and skilled individuals who have considerable expertise in the areas of honey bee biology, health, disease diagnosis, treatment, husbandry, apiary maintenance, pollination, and honey production. The credentials needed to become an apiary inspector are extensive, requiring not only an intimate knowledge of not only honey bees but also field training of the methods involved in beekeeping. Inspectors also must be educated in identifying, diagnosing, and treating honey bee health issues. The best apiary inspectors are those that not only possess this level of education and experience but also have a firm understanding of the complexities of a colony and the dynamics of the beekeeping community.

The primary duty and regulatory authority of an apiary inspector are performing routine or investigative health inspections of honey bee hives. These inspections could be for the purposes of routine annual evaluation, interstate or international transport, or investigation of a particular health issue. Regardless of the purpose, honey bee health inspections evaluate every aspect of both the individual colony (queen, brood, workers, drones, bee behavior, food stores, equipment condition, and so forth) and the apiary as a whole (location, setup, management, equipment storage, transport, and so forth). Inspectors may take samples for bacterial, fungal, viral, and arthropod pest diagnosis (**Figs. 3** and **4**). These samples either are analyzed internally, using local government or university diagnostic laboratories, or externally through submissions to federal or private laboratories (**Table 1**). The US Department of Agriculture (USDA) Agricultural Research Service (ARS) Bee Research Laboratory provides free honey bee disease and pest diagnostic services and is used by many apiary programs across the United States. Following an inspection, an apiary inspector issues a report providing the results along with any necessary supporting recommendations for treatment, management, or orders required to meet regulations.

If a health issue is detected during the inspection, the apiary inspector instructs and executes the treatment or decommission of the affected colony/colonies, if necessary. Most honey bee health issues can be treated using cultural methods, pesticides, proper feeding, or antibiotics. AFB is an exception to the rule given that it is extremely virulent and spreads readily between colonies. In most states, provinces, and territories, AFB detection in a hive requires depopulation of the hive followed by destruction, which can include burning of all infected material (discussed later) (**Figs. 5** and **6**). As previously described, many apiary programs were created in response to the spread and deleterious impact AFB had on honey bee colonies throughout North America. Through the efforts of these individual programs, AFB has been broadly suppressed. Although AFB is not commonly found these days, most apiary programs maintain regulatory authority for this disease. In many states, provinces, and territories, AFB is a reportable disease, meaning that beekeepers are required to inform their local apiary program if they have or suspect they have AFB in their operations.[2]

Like many other types of livestock, honey bees often require health certificates and other documentation before queens, colonies, or used equipment can be moved

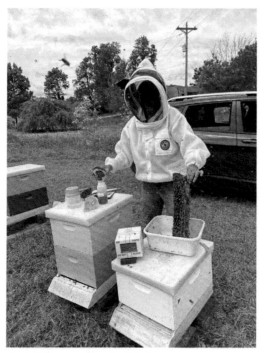

Fig. 3. Apiary inspector taking samples of adult bees.

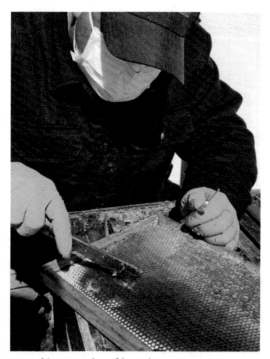

Fig. 4. Apiary inspector taking samples of brood.

Table 1
Honey bee diagnostic laboratory services for bacterial pathogens

			Pathogen		Sample		
Laboratory Name	Geographic Service Area	Location	American Foulbrood	European Foulbrood	Type	Fee	Analysis Type
USDA ARS Bee Research Laboratory	USA	Beltsville, MD	+	+	Brood	No	Culture
Utah Department of Agriculture and Food	USA	Salt Lake City, UT	+	+	Brood	Yes	PCR assay
North Carolina State University	USA	Raleigh, NC	+	+	Brood	Yes	Culture
National Agricultural Genotyping Center	USA	Fargo, ND	+	+	Brood, Adult bees	Yes	PCR
University of Guelph Animal Health Laboratory	Canada	Guelph, Ontario	+	+	Brood	Yes	Culture
Province of Manitoba Veterinary Diagnostic Services	Canada	Winnipeg, Manitoba	+	+	Brood, Adult bees	Yes	Culture, PCR
Grande Prairie Regional College National Bee Diagnostic Centre	Canada	Beaverlodge, Alberta	+	+	Brood, Adult bees	Yes	Culture, PCR
Clemson University	USA	Pendleton, South Carolina	+	+	Brood, Adult bees	Yes	PCR assay

Abbreviation: PCR, polymerase chain reaction. +, meaning lab offers this type of pathogen analysis.

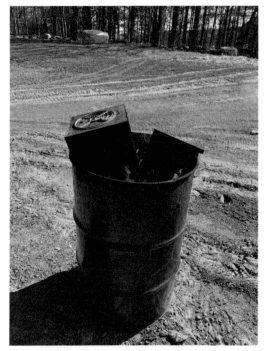

Fig. 5. Destruction of AFB, *Paenibacillus larvae*–infected nucleus hive.

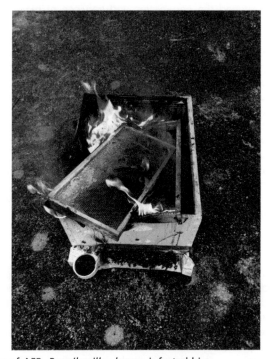

Fig. 6. Destruction of AFB, *Paenibacillus larvae*–infected hive.

between states, provinces, territories, and internationally. Inspectors issue health certificates and permits for interstate movement or international shipment, when requested by a beekeeper. These types of inspections often contain thousands of individual honey bee colonies, so health certificates often are issued based on an inspection of 5% to 20% of the total shipment.

In 1922, the federal Honey Bee Importation Act went into place that restricted the entry of some populations of honey bees into the United States from other countries.[6,7] At present, most states, territories, and provinces have laws and regulations relating to honey bees and beekeeping.[2,8] In general, the focus on these laws and regulations are specific to the occurrence, spread, mitigation, or treatment of honey bee diseases (AFB, EFB, and so forth) and associated invasive parasites or pests. Diseases, pests, and invasive organisms often are regulated in these laws and contain specific language regarding inspections, disease incidence, notification, treatment, and quarantine. Besides pest and disease language, many apiary laws also contain rules about interstate movement, entry of honey bee colonies, issuance of permits, or health certificates as well as state registration requirements and restrictions regarding the location of apiaries.

In addition to the regulatory component of these positions and programs, apiary inspectors also take on duties and perform services related to providing education, conducting or assisting with research projects, collaborating interdepartmentally to market the beekeeping industry, and providing laboratory diagnostic services of disease samples. Apiary programs tend to be multifaceted and dynamic, adapting to meet the needs of beekeepers under a framework of regulatory stewardship and a passion for healthy honey bees. Despite the need, these programs often are underfunded and understaffed, with many states, provinces, and territories possessing only a single individual or part-time apiary inspector. This limitation, combined with the increased interest in beekeeping, has stretched the capabilities and services of many apiary programs, potentially allowing for undetected incidences of infectious disease.

Apiary inspectors welcome a collaborative relationship with veterinarians who are interested in performing duties that support honey bee health and beekeepers through disease detection, diagnosis, and treatment. Given the regulatory authority of apiary inspectors and expertise of veterinarians, it is important to first establish a relationship and build a communication pathway. Veterinarians should familiarize themselves with the specific language of the laws and regulations for each state, province, and territory in which they work as well as those in surrounding jurisdictions. The best resource to find links to the laws, regulations, and local inspector is on the Apiary Inspectors of America[9] and Canadian Association of Professional Apiculturists[10] Web sites. Once this relationship has been established, the veterinarian should maintain open communication with the apiary inspector to notify the discovery of any regulated disease or pests, such as AFB or EFB, or invasive concerns, such as the Asian giant hornet (*Vespa mandarinia*) or the *Tropilaelaps* mites species.

DISCUSSION

Since the nineteenth century, commercial and migratory beekeepers largely have been marginalized by regulations from federal regulatory agencies, including the FDA and the Environmental Protection Agency (EPA). Since the 1950s, the commercial beekeeping industry has evolved hand-in-hand with industrial agriculture. As farms became larger, they required more honey bees for fruit and vegetable production, increasing the price paid per hive for pollination rentals. Beekeepers became accustomed to using antibiotics to suppress visible outbreaks of AFB, especially in the middle of pollination season. The list of crops that require pollination is long (at least 150 crops in North America), but the almond industry is considered the most critical because the seed-set required for a successful crop cannot happen with any other pollinator but honey bees.[11,12] Commercial beekeepers also use antibiotics to suppress visible AFB and EFB symptoms in the small nucleus colonies (commonly called "nucs") that are produced for sale to consumers.

These different and widespread uses of antibiotics led to their overuse. The first medications used by beekeepers were the sulfa drugs, namely sulfathiazole in the early 1950s.[13] Oxytetracycline (Terramycin), a broad-spectrum tetracycline, became available to beekeepers later in the 1950s, but due to its popularity beekeepers are starting to see resistance to this treatment. The antibiotic lincomycin (Lincomix) was introduced in the 1990s. Finally, in 2005, tylosin tartrate (Tylan) was approved for the control of AFB, but because beekeepers have to remove honey supers for a period of time with the use of this antibiotic, they prefer to use another method of control. Resistance to 1 or more of these antibiotics, such as Lincomix, has been shown in several AFB and EFB populations. Currently in Canada and the United States, there are only a few registered medications and pesticides available for use in honey bee hives.[14,15]

There has been some recent research at Brigham Young University focused on phages, which act as a virus to the AFB bacteria, but that research currently is ongoing and has yet to receive EPA approval.[16] Veterinarians are encouraged to read about this research so that they can stay current on the latest efforts for nonantibiotic control of AFB.

There are some practical tips for veterinarians as they learn more about beekeeping. There are AFB and EFB lateral flow quick diagnostic kits currently on the market that cost approximately $15.00 per kit (**Fig. 7**). These kits must be stored properly and, before use, expiration dates of the test kit should be checked. If a veterinarian notices clinical signs suggestive of AFB, such as a positive rope test or bad odor, the diagnostic quick kit can give a presumptive diagnosis in the field. False-negative results and false-positive results are possible, so all diagnoses should be laboratory confirmed. Veterinarians should consider carrying inventory of these test kits not only for use during clinical examinations but also as a source for beekeepers because access to local beekeeping vendors often is limited. This is a valuable service that veterinarians can provide.

If a veterinarian is called to do an inspection of an AFB hive, they should take a diagnostic kit, disposable gloves, a small flashlight, a shovel, and a can of lighter fluid. If a veterinarian wants to take a sample, with the permission of the beekeeper, they can collect a frame or a subsection of comb from the brood area and send the sample to 1 of the laboratories included in **Table 1**. If the colony is suspected to have or confirmed to have AFB, the veterinarian should notify the apiary inspector if the state has an apiary program.

Because antibiotics are not effective against AFB, the veterinarian and apiary inspector must work together in destroying the infected materials. For example, here are some basic directions on how to burn a positively identified AFB case. If possible, wait until the end of the day when all forager bees have returned before these steps are taken:

- Check all the other hives in the apiary for signs of AFB. Use a different hive tool from the one used to check the AFB-identified hive and change disposable gloves after every colony inspection.
- Ideally during the day, pour a 5-gallon bucket of soapy water into the hive from the top. This kills the bees while still allowing time for the equipment to dry out before burning.

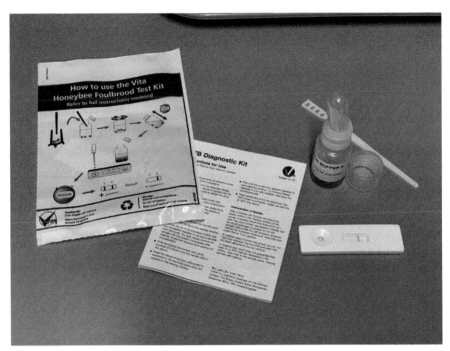

Fig. 7. Diagnostic field kit for testing suspect brood presenting symptoms for AFB, *Paenibacillus larvae*, or EFB, *Melissococcus plutonius*.

- Dig a pit or set up a burn barrel. If necessary, consult the local fire department and notify them of the intention to burn a diseased hive and double-check if any burn bans are in place.
- Start a fire with the diseased frames in the pit or burn barrel first, saving the boxes for last. Make sure that the fire does not get out of control before adding more bee equipment (supers, lid, inner cover, and base). Always have a fire extinguisher and several 5-gallon buckets of water on hand.
- Once the hive has been burned, cover the pit or put out the fire in the barrel.
- If a burn ban is in place and burning is not allowed, put all materials into black plastic bags, seal, and then transport to local landfill for disposal.

If a hive has EFB, most states, provinces, and territories do not require burning. If the EFB disease has spread to other hives, the veterinarian may need to issue a VFD to the beekeeper.[17]

As veterinarians become more familiar with the beekeeping community and honey bee biology, they can assist with hive health by offering additional diagnostic services, such as *Varroa* mite sampling and *Nosema* detection. Veterinarians also may find a place for their leadership if their state has a Managed Pollinator Protection Plan (MP3). Prior to the 2017 VFD enacted by the FDA, the EPA advised states to develop an MP3 to be tailored to each state's unique geography and beekeeping priorities.[18] These plans often prioritize hive health by encouraging farmers and landowners (including homeowners) to reduce chemical use or, if necessary, to communicate with beekeepers prior to application. But there are other components to the MP3 as well, depending on the state in question. Many MP3s have best management practices defined by a state's division of environmental services offices. Veterinarians should reach out to the apiary program and/or the state department of agriculture to obtain the most recent copy of the state MP3, keeping in mind that states see these plans as evolving and not static documents. No 2 MP3s are the same. Some states do not have a plan at all. Other states want to include all pollinators, not just managed pollinators, such as honey bees. In other words, there are multiple ways that veterinarians can be involved in a state's pollinator issues, not just from a medical standpoint.

Multiple actions can help improve proficiency in honey bee veterinary medicine. Establish a relationship with the state or provincial apiary inspector and arrange a time and place to meet at a beehive. Subscribe to the trade journals *American Bee Journal* or *Bee Culture* or both for a year. Join a local bee association and make an introduction as a veterinarian willing to be available in case there is a problem with a bee hive. Spend a year learning what is a "normal" brood, learn the flowers in the area, learn about winter clusters, and, importantly, learn what is abnormal for a honey bee colony and its inhabitants. Veterinarians often have to adapt to animals for which veterinary school did not prepare them. At the time of this writing, honey bees are one of these species of animals; they are fascinating in terms of sheer ingenuity. Aristotle once said that "beekeeping is farming for intellectuals," so veterinarians already are well-qualified to engage in this journey, hand-in-hand with apiary inspectors.

SUMMARY

Prior to the 2017 VFD, there were strict divisions between veterinarians and apiary inspectors. Now there is an opportunity for veterinary medicine and apiculture to intersect at a critical time when professional expertise will help ease the transition. The migratory beekeeping and honey production industry are more important, and arguably more reliant on antibiotics, than ever. The more informed and collaborative veterinarians and apiary inspectors are as professionals, the better able they will be to maintain healthy, viable honey bee hives for a thriving sustainable agricultural economy.

CLINICS CARE POINTS

- Become familiar with honey bee biology, field diagnosis, and disease management techniques.
- Communicate with an apiary inspector and become familiar with the laws, rules, and regulations for the municipalities in the local area.
- Cases of AFB require detection, clinical diagnosis, and laboratory confirmation.
- Contact a local apiary inspector when AFB is suspected and work together to manage the situation.

DISCLOSURE

The authors have nothing to disclose.

REFERENCES

1. Matthews WA, Sumner DA, Hanon T. Contributions of the U.S. honey industry to the U.S. economy 2018. Available at: https://aic.ucdavis.edu/wp-content/uploads/2019/02/HONEY-COMPLETE-DRAFT_FEBRUARY-11-2019.pdf. Assessed November 24, 2020.

2. Knox DA, Shimanuki H. In: Morse RA, Flottum K, editors. Honey bee pests, pred-ators, and diseases. 3rd edition. UK: Northern Bee Books; 2013. Appendix Seven.

3. Reed M, Caron DM, Rogers D. Honey Bee Health Coalition: identifying and miti-gating foulbrood in honey bee colonies and reducing the use of antibiotics – In-formation for beekeepers and veterinarians. 2020. Available at: https://honeybeehealthcoalition.org/foulbrood/. Accessed November 14, 2020.

4. U.S. Food and Drug Administration. Fact sheet: veterinary feed directive final rule and next steps. 2017. Available at: https://www.fda.gov/animal-veterinary/development-approval-process/fact-sheet-veterinary-feed-directive-final-rule-and-next-steps. Assessed November 24, 2020.

5. Health Canada. Food and drugs act: regulations amending the food and regula-tions (veterinary drugs antimicrobial resistance) 2017. Available at: https://gazette.gc.ca/rp-pr/p2/2017/2017-05-17/html/sor-dors76-eng.html. Assessed February 20, 2020.

6. Honey bee importation, U.S. Code § 7-281 (1922).

7. Shimanuki H, Lima P. In: Morse RA, Flottum K, editors. Honey bee pests, preda-tors, and diseases. 3rd edition. UK: Northern Bee Books; 2013. Appendix Six.

8. Apiary Inspectors of America. Laws and regulations. 2020. Available at: https://apiaryinspectors.org/. Accessed November 14, 2020.

9. Apiary Inspectors of America. Inspection services. 2020. Available at: https://apiaryinspectors.org/inspection-services/. Accessed November 14, 2020.

10. Canadian Association of Professional Apiculturists. 2020. Available at: https://capabees.com/. Accessed November 14, 2020.

11. Ferrier PM, Rucker RR, Thurman WN, et al. Economic effects and responses to changes in honey bee health, ERR-246. Washington, D.C: U.S. Department of Agriculture, Economic Research Service; 2018.

12. United States Department of Agriculture. Pollinators. 2020. Available at: https://www.usda.gov/pollinators. Accessed November 14, 2020.

13. Genersch E. American Foulbrood in honey bees and its causative agent, Paeni-bacillus larvae. J Invertebr Pathol 2010;103:S10–9.

14. Honey Bee Health Coalition. Registered medications and pesticides for honey bee health in the United States. 2020. Available at: https://honeybeehealthcoalition.org/wp-content/uploads/2020/10/HBHC_Approved_Medications_US_092320.pdf. Accessed November 14, 2020.

15. Honey Bee Health Coalition. Registered medications and pesticides for honey bee health in Canada. 2020. Available at: https://honeybeehealthcoalition.org/wp-content/uploads/2020/10/HBHC_Approved_Medications_Canada_092320.pdf. Accessed November 14, 2020.

16. Brady TS, Merrill BD, Hilton JA, et al. Bacteriophages as an alternative to conven-tional antibiotic use for the prevention or treatment of Paenibacillus larvae in hon-eybee hives. J Invertebr Pathol 2017;150:94–100.

17. Honey Bee Health Coalition. Identifying and mitigating foulbrood in honey bee colonies. 2020. Available at: https://honeybeehealthcoalition.org/foulbrood/. Ac-cessed November 14, 2020.

18. United States Environmental Protection Agency. Protecting bees and other polli-nators from pesticides. 2020. Available at: https://www.epa.gov/pollinator-protection. Accessed November 14, 2020.

Epidemiology and Biosecurity for Veterinarians Working with Honey bees (*Apis mellifera*)

Britteny Kyle, DVM[a],*, Katie Lee, MS, PhD[b], Stephen F. Pernal, PhD[c]

KEYWORDS

- Epidemiology • Biosecurity • Honey bee health management • Population medicine

KEY POINTS

- The principles of epidemiology and biosecurity can be applied to honey bees.
- There are currently several epidemiologic-based surveys going on in the United States and Canada.
- Veterinarians can work with beekeepers in the area of biosecurity to improve animal identification, traceability, and record keeping, and to reduce disease transmission.

INTRODUCTION

Honey bee veterinary medicine is a new and developing field in North America with veterinarians now responsible for the oversight of antimicrobial use in honey bee colonies. Although there are many differences between honey bees and the traditional food animal species under veterinary purview, the fundamental principles of epidemiology and biosecurity are largely the same.

Veterinarians working with honey bees will most often work at the colony level to examine, diagnose, and treat honey bee pests and diseases. The colony can be viewed as the patient, and the veterinarian can sample the individual honey bees, either as adults or as a brood, to inform clinical decisions. When applying herd health management practices, veterinarians will work at the apiary level, with colonies within the apiary being analogous to a herd. In large beekeeping operations, veterinarians may consider all colonies within the operation to be the herd, with the individual apiaries being analogous to pens of animals.

[a] Department of Population Medicine, Ontario Veterinary College, University of Guelph, 50 Stone Road East, Guelph, Ontario N1G 2W1, Canada; [b] University of Minnesota Extension, 1980 Folwell Avenue, Suite 219, Saint Paul, MN, USA; [c] Agriculture and Agri-Food Canada, Beaverlodge Research Farm, PO Box 29, Beaverlodge, Alberta T0H 0C0, Canada
* Corresponding author.
E-mail address: kyleb@uoguelph.ca

Vet Clin Food Anim 37 (2021) 479–490
https://doi.org/10.1016/j.cvfa.2021.06.004
0749-0720/21/Crown Copyright © 2021 Published by Elsevier Inc. All rights reserved.
vetfood.theclinics.com

The veterinary needs of the client will differ with the type of beekeeping operation. There are three main types of beekeeping operations: hobbyists, side-liners, and commercial. In general, hobbyists own anywhere from 1 to 50 colonies, and the motivation for keeping bees is as a hobby. Most hobby beekeepers maintain their colonies in one location year-round. In contrast, commercial beekeepers manage hundreds or even thousands of colonies with most or all of their income derived from beekeeping. Commercial operations generate income through several avenues, including pollination services; livestock supply, such as queens, package bees, and nucleus colonies; and the sale of hive products, such as honey or pollen. Commercial beekeepers are often migratory, moving their bees to different locations based on the bloom phenology of plants or crops to produce honey or to pollinate agriculturally important commodities. Commercial operations typically keep around 40 colonies in a single apiary and occasionally keep hundreds or thousands of colonies in a "holding yard" for very short periods of time. In between hobbyists and commercial beekeepers are the side-liners. This group typically owns 50 to a few hundred colonies. Side-liners earn some income from beekeeping but it may not be their primary income source. Some side-liner beekeepers are migratory. Veterinarians should strive to understand the scale of the beekeeping operation as well as the reason for keeping bees.

Honey bees present many challenges to biosecurity. Although honey bees prefer to forage close to their hive, they have been shown to fly up to 12 km (8 miles) for high-profit forage.[1] While on foraging flights, worker honey bees will collect 1 of 4 things: nectar, pollen, water, or propolis, from the environment. Unlike with many of our other food animal species, beekeepers cannot control where the bees forage for food or water, nor what they interact with while outside the hive. Honey bees are affected by bacterial, fungal, and viral pathogens, and parasites, most notably *Varroa destructor*. These pathogens and parasites can spread from bee to bee within a colony and among colonies by drifting and robbing bees. Despite these challenges, biosecurity standards can still be used.

DISCUSSION OF EPIDEMIOLOGY

Epidemiology is the study of the distribution and determinants of states of health, including disease, within a population.[2] The application of epidemiology to honey bees follows the same principles and is equally as important as in other veterinary species.

The population of honey bees being evaluated for disease must be defined. The population may be the national herd, the managed colonies within a state or province, or at a more local level. Populations can also be defined based on type of beekeeping operation or services provided, such as the migratory population that travels within or out of state/province for pollination purposes. Honey bee populations are typically open. Additions commonly occur through the purchase of nucleus colonies or package bees, the capture of swarms, and colony splits.[3] The epidemiologic unit under study for honey bees could be the individual honey bees, the colonies, the apiary, or the beekeeping operation.[3]

Establishing measures of disease frequency in honey bees allows for monitoring changes in disease levels and the evaluation of disease mitigation strategies. Measures of disease frequency can be carried out at all levels of the honey bee population. Apparent prevalence of disease among colonies will depend largely on clinical expression of the disease and the ability of the beekeeper, apiary inspector, researcher, or veterinarian to detect it as well as the sensitivity and specificity of the diagnostic tests used.[3] Incidence is another measure that is commonly used, with the time period often established as a season, such as the winter for annual winter colony-loss surveys.[3,4]

Transmission pathways of the various honey bee pests and diseases are important for the veterinarian to understand. As with all other species, transmission can occur either horizontally or vertically. However, in honey bees, the transmission can occur both within and between colonies.[5]

Intracolony transmission of pathogens and pests occurs horizontally from a worker to another adult bee or to the developing brood. Horizontal intracolony transmission can also occur via vectors, mainly by the parasitic mite V destructor, which has been shown to transmit deformed wing virus (DWV),[6,7] slow paralysis virus (SPV),[6] and Israeli acute paralysis virus (IAPV),[8] and evidence has suggested it may also be a mechanical or biological vector of several other viruses, including sacbrood virus (SBV),[7,9] acute bee paralysis virus (ABPV),[7] Kashmir bee virus (KBV),[9,10] and chronic bee paralysis virus (CBPV).[11] Some viral pathogens can also be transmitted vertically within the colony when spread from the queen to her offspring.[5,9]

Intercolony horizontal transmission of pathogens and pests occurs with drifting, robbing, contact during foraging, mechanical and biological vectors (mainly V destructor), through fomites, and with beekeeper activities.[5] For example, water contaminated with feces from a bee with the microsporidian parasite Nosema apis or Nosema ceranae can infect drinking bees.[12] Viruses, Nosema spp, and V destructor mites can be passed to other bees at flowers.[13–15] Beekeeper activities that can lead to intercolony horizontal transmission include exchanging equipment and frames of bees between colonies, and feeding of honey to other colonies. Vertical intercolony transmission occurs during swarming when half of the honey bees and the original queen leave to establish a new colony and potentially take disease or parasites with them.[5]

Veterinarians can work with beekeepers to reduce both intracolony and intercolony transmission. During clinical examination (inspection), care must be taken to handle the bees in such a way as to reduce the risk of crushing bees, which can increase intracolony horizontal transmission.[5] Sugar syrup feeders used inside the colony should have a floater or ladder to reduce bees drowning in, and consequently contaminating, the feed that other bees in the colony are consuming. For intercolony horizontal transmission, drifting can be significant in managed situations with a high density of colonies.[5,16] Beekeepers often determine their apiary stocking rate by available floral resources in the local environment. However, the recommended stocking density of the apiary to reduce drifting depends on the landmarks in the local environment as well as the layout and visual differentiation of the colonies within the bee yard. Well-spaced visually distinct hives in a nonlinear conformation is recommended to reduce drifting.[17,18] In high-density commercial operations, treating the entire apiary collectively as one unit can be important to manage the disease and pest loads of the herd and reduce intercolony transmission. Robbing is another aspect of horizontal intercolony transmission that can be reduced with proper management. Colonies weakened by pests and diseases are susceptible to robbing events, and the bees from the healthy, robbing colony can pick up those pests and diseases.[19] The best defense against robbing is to keep strong, healthy colonies. Strong colonies, however, are more likely to engage in robbing behavior and may be at greater risk of acquiring pathogens and pests. Veterinarians and their beekeeper clients should ensure that colonies are kept strong, of equal strength to other colonies within the apiary, and inspected regularly for evidence of pests and diseases. During a forage dearth, entrance reducers should be used to decrease the area that the guard bees need to defend against robbing bees. After a dearth, inspections should be done to look for evidence of disease transmission. Furthermore, veterinarians should be mindful to limit inspections during a dearth, as this can trigger robbing behavior. Any colonies that have died, commonly referred to as dead-outs, should be removed from the apiary as quickly as possible to prevent robbing of the hive. A common method of supplemental feeding is barrel, or rob feeding, in which an open container of sugar syrup is placed in the apiary. Although this feeding method is less labor intensive, it increases the risk of intercolony disease transmission within and between nearby apiaries. Other management practices, such as transferring frames to another colony or moving bees between colonies, can increase the risk of horizontal transmission and should be advised against where possible.[5] Areas with a high density of beekeepers with varying management practices, such as is commonly found in urban environments, are at greater risk of intercolony disease transmission.

From a clinical perspective, veterinarians need to know how many bees within a colony to sample to accurately determine the disease status of the colony. For example, it is recommended to check a sample of 300 adult bees collected from a frame with brood to determine the infestation level of the parasitic mite V destructor.[20] Diagnostic laboratories normally offer guidelines for minimum sample size submission depending on what is being sampled and for which test. It is also important to know how many colonies within an apiary need to be sampled to determine the disease status at the apiary level. Using the example of V destructor, it has been shown that sampling 8 colonies within an apiary provides an estimate of the infestation level within the apiary that can be used to inform a management decision.[20] Veterinarians are encouraged to work with the beekeeper, their state/provincial apiary program, and the diagnostic laboratory to develop a suitable sampling plan for the various pests and diseases of interest.

There are currently several programs in the United States and Canada that collect epidemiologic information on honey bees (**Table 1**). Annual colony monitoring surveys are done on the national level in both countries. The Canadian Association of Provincial Apiculturists has collected and disseminated information on annual colony losses in Canada since 2007.[21] This collection and dissemination of information is done through coordinated survey administration by the Provincial Apiary programs in order to collect and present information on the national population.[21] Information collected includes total colony counts, winter mortalities, beekeeper perception on the cause of winter losses, and management practices regarding V destructor, Nosema spp, and American foulbrood (AFB).[21] In addition to this program, the National Honey Bee Health Survey was performed by cooperation of industry, the National Bee Diagnostic Centre, governmental partners, and academia from 2014 to 2017.[22] This survey began in Alberta and Manitoba, but expanded each year to become representative of the national honey bee herd.[22] Data collected came from visual inspections for disease, pests, and the status of the queen as well as apiary-level samples pooled from 10 randomly selected colonies within each apiary. Samples were analyzed for AFB (including checking for resistance to antimicrobials), European foulbrood (EFB), nosema, V destructor mites, tracheal mites, the presence of exotic pests, numerous viruses (ABPV, black queen cell virus, CBPV, DWV, IAPV, KBV, SBV, Lake Sinai virus, and SPV), hybridization with Africanized honey bees, and chemical residues in bee bread.[22] In the United States, annual monitoring on the national level is performed by the US Department of Agriculture (USDA) Animal Plant Health Inspection Service (APHIS) in collaboration with the University of Maryland, USDA Agricultural Research Service, and the State Apiary Inspection programs.[23] Surveying is done in conjunction with the Bee Informed Partnership, which is discussed in more detail below. The USDA APHIS National Honey Bee Disease Survey has 3 objectives: monitoring for the presence of exotic threats, evaluation of honey bee health, and longitudinal monitoring for pests and diseases.[23] Longitudinal monitoring involves volunteer states to sample 5

Table 1
Summary of surveillance efforts in Canada and the United States

Group	Country	Survey of Colony Losses	Survey of Management Practices	Efforts		
				Single Time Point Monitoring of Current Diseases and Parasites	Single Time Point Monitoring of Exotic Diseases and Parasites	Longitudinal Monitoring of Diseases and Parasites
Canadian Association of Provincial Apiculturists (CAPA)	Canada	X	X			
Provincial Apiary Program	Canada	X	X	X		
National Honey Bee Health Survey	Canada			X	X	X
USDA Animal Plant Health Inspection Service (APHIS)	United States			X	X	X
Bee Informed Partnership	United States	X	X	X		X
State Apiary Inspection	United States			X		

Types of honey bee population surveillance efforts performed by programs in Canada and the United States. These programs may be of interest to veterinarians that are developing a colony-monitoring program or are interested in current trends of honey bee health.

beekeepers once in the spring and once in the fall for the presence of several pests, diseases, and pesticide residues as well as the collection of management information and annual colony mortalities.[23] These data are used to determine the seasonality of pests and disease as well as evaluation over time, which allows for the potential identification of correlations between seasonal distribution patterns and colony losses.[23] Overall, the annual survey analyzes samples for the presence of the foreign parasitic mite *Tropilaelaps*, *Apis cerana* (a species of honey bee native to the Asian continent), *V destructor*, *Nosema* spp, and numerous viruses.[23] Furthermore, visual inspection is done to check for several diseases, such as AFB, EFB, chalkbrood, viruses, and pests, such as small hive beetle and wax moths.[23] Bee bread is analyzed for 199 different pesticide residues.[23] In addition to the surveys, both countries have national bee laboratories, as well as numerous local laboratories that carry out testing on honey bees.

The health of honey bee populations is evaluated at the provincial/state level through the Apiary Inspection Programs. The inspection programs are largely, although not exclusively, focused on AFB, caused by the etiologic agent *Paenibacillus larvae*, but may also include other pests and diseases that vary based on the needs of the individual states and provinces. More information about the state and provincial apiary programs is discussed in another article in this issue.

In the United States, the Bee Informed Partnership is a nonprofit organization known for their epidemiologic work through many annual projects. The honey bee colony loss survey queries beekeepers about colony mortality during both the winter and the active beekeeping season, beekeepers' perceived reason for colony losses, *V destructor* monitoring and treatment/management practices, supplemental feeding practices, queen management, and other management practices regarding treatment protocols, comb, dead-outs, and replacement colonies.[24] The Sentinel Apiary Program is a fee-based program for beekeepers that want to monitor colonies monthly for *V destructor* and *Nosema* levels, with an option to track hive weight with the use of a hive scale.[24] The Bee Informed Partnership also collaborates in the MiteCheck colony monitoring program whereby beekeepers across Canada, the United States, and Mexico are invited to report *V destructor* levels in order to develop a map showing the location of participants sampling for this parasite.[24] Tech-Transfer Teams (based on the Canadian concept) work with commercial beekeepers to monitor disease and pests, occasionally longitudinally.[24] Tech-Transfer Teams are also present in many Canadian provinces, often as part of the provincial beekeepers' organizations, and work on disease monitoring, research, education, and information dissemination to beekeepers.

These programs, whether national or more local, are important for monitoring and evaluating honey bee health at the population level. Veterinarians are encouraged to learn about the programs carried out in their respective locations. There may be opportunities for veterinarians and respective beekeeper clients to become involved, and these programs also provide information that is useful for veterinarians interested in understanding historical and current trends in honey bee health.

DISCUSSION OF BIOSECURITY

A fundamental aspect of biosecurity is identification of the colonies within an operation. Identifying the colonies is required for traceability, which is important not only for biosecurity but also for food safety so that honey can be traced back to the source apiary (more information on food safety practices for honey production can be found in the Canadian Bee Industry Safety Quality Traceability Producer Manual published by the Canadian Honey Council[25]). Beekeepers may not have a formal identification system in place. It is recommended that veterinarians work with the beekeeper to develop a permanent unique identifier that is logical and easy for the beekeeper to implement. Challenges include the ability to withstand exposure to the elements, the swapping of boxes and frames of bees between colonies, retiring or changing a label at colony death, and the mobile nature of migratory operations. In small operations, paint color or a number recorded on the hive boxes may be feasible (**Fig. 1**). Larger operations, and particularly migratory ones, may benefit from the use of livestock ear tags or radiofrequency identification tags attached to hive boxes. In addition to identifying the hive, and subsequently the colony within it, beekeepers should also have a way to identify and differentiate the apiaries, or bee yards, such as with street address or GPS coordinates. Within the colony, queens can be identified with a colored dot on the dorsal thorax following the international queen bee color marking code to allow for quick identification, age determination, recognition of queen events, such as supersedure and swarming, and when combined with good record keeping, traceability.[26,27]

Veterinarians must keep complete medical records for any work done on honey bee patients. It is also advisable for the beekeeper to have a good record-keeping system in place. Current record systems used may be simplistic, such as placing a rock on top of a colony to identify that something was or needs to be done, or notes written on the inside or outside of the hive lid with permanent marker or a lumber crayon (**Fig. 2**). More formal record-keeping systems may include paper notes, yard books dedicated to each apiary, or computerized databases with data entry hive-side on a laptop or mobile device. The best record-keeping system to use will vary with the type and

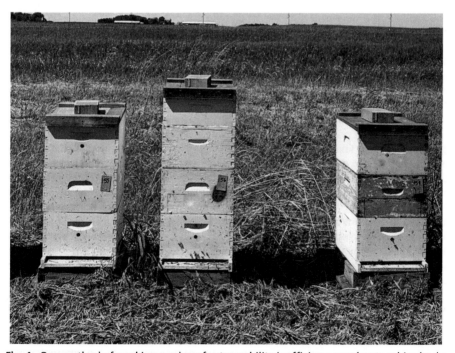

Fig. 1. One method of marking a colony for traceability is affixing a number to a hive body. An example is stapling a plastic card with a colony number written in paint pen. Other information can be included on the card, like the month the colony was sampled.

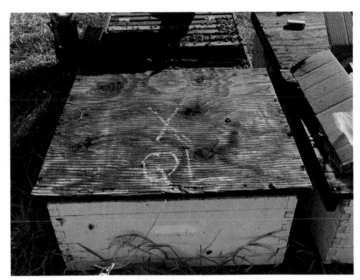

Fig. 2. A common way beekeepers record management notes in the apiary is by writing on the lid with a permanent marker or lumber crayon. Here, the colony was queenless, which is indicated by writing "QL" as shorthand.

size of the beekeeping operation. Key components should include ease of use, ability to record detailed information, easy retrieval of data, and long-term storage ability. A good resource of record templates on all different aspects of beekeeping, including colony assessment and disease monitoring and treatment, is the Canadian Beekeepers' Practical Handbook to Bee Biosecurity and Food Safety prepared by the Canadian Honey Council.[28]

Veterinarians need to take biosecurity precautions during hive inspections, particularly when evaluating weak or sick colonies. Without proper protocols, disease can be spread between colonies and apiaries during inspection. It is recommended that veterinarians wear nitrile gloves when handling bees, and these gloves should be changed between colonies and especially after working in sick hives. Any suspect diseased colonies should be examined last. Tools are a potential vehicle for spreading pathogens. Ideally, the veterinarian will use the beekeeper's tools. Metal tools can be disinfected between colonies by scraping clean and then placing in a lit smoker and pumping the bellows a few times or scorching with a blow torch.[18] Alternatively, tools can be scraped of debris and sprayed or scrubbed with a bleach solution. Bleach, however, in concentrations commonly available and in the presence of organic material, may be insufficient to kill spores of *P larvae* (AFB).[29] It is important to keep the apiary clean at all times. Any honey or sugar syrup spills that happen during inspection should be cleaned immediately, and hive debris and dead bees should be properly disposed of. Fomite transmission is possible between apiaries on bee suits, boots, and vehicles. Wherever possible, suits should be changed and boots cleaned between bee yards. At a minimum, this needs to be done between visits to different operations.

When a sick colony is discovered, steps should be taken to reduce the risk of intercolony transmission. If a reportable or notifiable disease is part of the differential list, such as AFB, the proper authorities need to be consulted before any further handling or treatment of the colony. In cases of nonnotifiable/nonreportable diseases from which the colony may recover, ideally the colony can be quarantined. Quarantine apiaries should be isolated from other apiary locations, ideally at a distance to reduce the likelihood of flight overlap. Care must be taken when moving a colony to prevent contamination of the environment and the vehicle. Colonies should be moved when foragers are inside the hive and not out flying (eg, early morning or late in the day). When a separate quarantine yard is not feasible, yet the colony is to be treated, it may still be beneficial to quarantine the sick colony within the apiary when the disease is not highly transmissible or virulent; this would involve having dedicated equipment and tools for use only in the sick colony.[30]

Veterinarians need to consider the cost of implementing protocols relative to the cost of not intervening. Performing a cost-benefit analysis may be of particular importance to commercial beekeeping operations. The cost of a prevention or treatment can be weighed against the cost to replace a colony that is lost to the disease of interest. Replacement costs are not only the cost of the bees to establish a new colony and perhaps new equipment but also the inputs, mainly time and feed supplementation, that it takes to establish a colony of equal size and productivity as to the one lost.[3] Not intervening, however, could lead to an issue that persists for years with economic and welfare consequences. Consideration should also be given to culling sick colonies. Culling is the best way to prevent the spread of pathogens between colonies and can be paired with the destruction of equipment in cases whereby the pathogen can be spread through contaminated comb. It may be more economical to cull the colony, including the potential destruction of equipment, compared with the cost of treatment and risk of transmission to other colonies. Equipment, including wax comb, can be sterilized using ozone or at an irradiation facility. However, the logistics, cost of services, and transportation may be prohibitive. Veterinarians must be aware of state/provincial legislation regarding reporting and management of honey bee pests and diseases, particularly the bacterial disease AFB.

Biosecurity protocols around beekeeping equipment is an area where veterinarians can work with beekeepers to make improvements. It is common practice to purchase used beekeeping equipment, such as hive bodies and frames, as it is often less expensive. Used equipment also requires less energy and time, as the bees do not need to draw out all new comb. Used equipment, however, comes with the significant risk of being contaminated with pathogens and chemical residues and should be advised against. In cases when used equipment is purchased, it should be sterilized (ie, irradiated) before use and in some locations may be required to have a permit allowing its sale.[18] In addition to the purchase of used equipment, beekeepers may wish to reuse equipment in which a colony has died (ie, a dead-out). Necropsies should be performed to determine cause of death, and frames of comb should not be reused unless the cause is determined to be nonpathogenic in nature. Other hive components from dead-outs should be thoroughly cleaned and sterilized (by scorching, wax dipping, or irradiation) before reuse. All equipment should be regularly inspected to ensure it is in good working condition, and that there are no visible signs of disease, such as AFB scale. It is recommended that beekeepers have a systematic way to ensure a regular turnover of frames. Research by Berry and Delaplane[31] showed that there were health and reproductive benefits to being housed on new comb. Frames can be branded with the year they are installed and 20% to 30% of frames culled each year for a 3- to 5-year turnover, as is currently recommended in the industry.[26,32]

Supplemental feeding is a common practice among beekeepers, and when not done properly can allow for the introduction and transmission of pathogens. It has been demonstrated that both honey and pollen can be contaminated with spores of *P larvae* (the etiologic agent of AFB), *N apis*, *N ceranae*, and *Ascosphaera apis* (the etiologic agent of chalkbrood).[33] Honey should not be fed back to colonies, especially if the donor colony cannot be guaranteed to be free of disease.[18] Similarly, pollen should only be collected from colonies demonstrated to be free of disease or purchased from reputable sources that ensure it is disease-free, possibly by irradiation.[18] As discussed above, care needs to be taken in the administration of supplemental feed to prevent disease transmission within and between colonies.

Veterinarians are encouraged to learn about biosecurity standards specific to the beekeeping industry. In Canada, the Canadian Food Inspection Agency (CFIA) developed the National Bee Farm-Level Biosecurity Standard with information relevant to anyone keeping or working with honey bees, leafcutter bees, and bumble bees.[34] There is also a corresponding Honey Bee Biosecurity Checklist.[35] Both documents can be found online on the CFIA Web site (https://inspection.gc.ca).

SUMMARY

Currently veterinarians in Canada and the United States are only tasked with oversight of the use of antimicrobials in apiculture. Veterinary training, however, can be applied to honey bees just as in other food animal species. Veterinarians are encouraged to learn about apiculture, including current disease-monitoring programs, biosecurity standards, and legislation and regulations specific to the state or province where they are licensed to practice.

CLINICS CARE POINTS

- There is no one-size-fits-all answer; veterinarians need to work *with* the beekeeper to come up with solutions that work for the given operation.
- Biosecurity is an area that veterinarians are well trained in, and they can apply their expertise from other animal species.
- Changing practices, such as identification of colonies and record keeping, will take time. Set goals with the client and work toward them.
- Demonstration that the recommended practices save beekeepers time and expense in the long run will help with acceptance and implementation.

DISCLOSURE

The authors have nothing to disclose.

REFERENCES

1. Beekman M, Ratnieks FLW. Long-range foraging by the honey-bee, *Apis mellifera* L. Funct Ecol 2000;14:490–6.
2. Porta MS, International Epidemiological Association. A dictionary of epidemiology. Vol 5th edition. Edited for the International Epidemiological Association by Miquel Porta; associate editors. Oxford University Press; 2008. Available at: http://web.a.ebscohost.com.subzero.lib.uoguelph.ca/ehost/ebookviewer/ebook/ZTAwMHhuYV9fMzE1MzM2X19BTg2?sid=98c38270-2834-448c-8c25-61a709b20ef7@sdc-v-sessmgr02&vid=0&format=EB&rid=1. Accessed December 26, 2020.

3. vanEngelsdorp D, Lengerich E, Spleen A, et al. Standard epidemiological methods to understand and improve *Apis mellifera* health. J Apicultural Res 2013;52(4):1–16.

4. Lee K, Steinhauer N, Travis DA, et al. Honey bee surveillance: a tool for understanding and improving honey bee health. Curr Opin Insect Sci 2015;10:37–44.

5. Fries I, Camazine S. Implications of horizontal and vertical pathogen transmission for honey bee epidemiology. Apidologie 2001;32(3):199–214.

6. Santillán-Galicia T, Ball BV, Clark SJ, et al. Transmission of deformed wing virus and slow paralysis virus to adult bees (*Apis mellifera* L.) by *Varroa destructor*. J Apicultural Res 2010;49(2):141–8.

7. Tentcheva D, Gauthier L, Zappulla N, et al. Prevalence and seasonal variations of six bee viruses in *Apis mellifera* L. and *Varroa destructor* mite populations in France. Appl Environ Microbiol 2004;70(12):7185–91.

8. Di Prisco G, Pennacchio F, Caprio E, et al. *Varroa destructor* is an effective vector of Israeli acute paralysis virus in the honey bee, *Apis mellifera*. J Gen Virol 2011; 92(1). https://doi.org/10.1099/vir.0.023853-0.

9. Shen M, Cui L, Ostiguy N, et al. Intricate transmission routes and interactions between picorna-like viruses (Kashmir bee virus and sacbrood virus) with the honey bee host and the parasitic varroa mite. J Gen Virol 2005;86(8). https://doi.org/10.1099/vir.0.80824-0.

10. Shen M, Yang X, Cox-Foster D, et al. The role of varroa mites in infections of Kashmir bee virus (KBV) and deformed wing virus (DWV) in honey bees. Virology 2005;342(1):141–9.

11. Celle O, Blanchard P, Olivier V, et al. Detection of chronic bee paralysis virus (CBPV) genome and its replicative RNA form in various hosts and possible ways of spread. Virus Res 2008;133(2):280–4.

12. Goblirsch M. *Nosema ceranae* disease of the honey bee (Apis mellifera). Apidologie 2018;49(1):131–50.

13. Higes M, Martín-Hernández R, Garrido-Bailon E, et al. Detection of infective *Nosema ceranae* (Microsporidia) spores in corbicular pollen of forager honey bees. J Invertebr Pathol 2008;97(1):76–8.

14. Peck DT, Smith ML, Seeley TD. *Varroa destructor* mites can nimbly climb from flowers onto foraging honey bees. PLoS One 2016;11(12):e0167798.

15. Mazzei M, Carrozza ML, Luisi E, et al. Infectivity of DWV associated to flower pollen: experimental evidence of a horizontal transmission route. PLoS One 2014; 9(11):e113448.

16. Seeley TD, Smith ML. Crowding honey bee colonies in apiaries can increase their vulnerability to the deadly ectoparasite *Varroa destructor*. Apidologie 2015;46(6): 716–27.

17. Dynes TL, Berry JA, Delaplane KS, et al. Reduced density and visually complex apiaries reduce parasite load and promote honey production and overwintering survival in honey bees. PLoS One 2019;14(5). https://doi.org/10.1371/journal.pone.0216286.

18. Eccles L, Kempers M, Gonzalez RM, et al. Canadian best management practices for honey bee health. Canada: Minister of Agriculture and Agri-Food; 2017.

19. Peck DT, Seeley TD. Mite bombs or robber lures? The roles of drifting and robbing in *Varroa destructor* transmission from collapsing honey bee colonies to their neighbors. PLoS One 2019;14(6):e0218392.

20. Lee KV, Moon RD, Burkness EC, et al. Practical sampling plans for *Varroa destructor* (Acari: Varroidae) in *Apis mellifera* (Hymenoptera: Apidae) colonies and apiaries. J Econ Entomol 2010;103(4):1039–50.

21. Annual Colony Loss Reports. Canadian Association of Provincial Apiculturists. 2020. Available at: https://capabees.com/capa-statement-on-honey-bees/; https://capabees.com/capa-statement-on-honey-bees/. Accessed January 17, 2021.
22. Grand Prairie Regional College. National Honey Bee Health Survey. Available at: https://www.gprc.ab.ca/research/initiatives/current/nat_survey.html. Accessed May 8, 2021.
23. Survey of Honey Bee Pests and Diseases. USDA animal and plant health inspection service 2020. Available at: https://www.aphis.usda.gov/aphis/ourfocus/planthealth/plant-pest-and-disease-programs/honey-bees/survey. Accessed January 17, 2021.
24. Bee Informed Project. 2020. Available at: https://beeinformed.org/. Accessed December 27, 2020.
25. Canadian Honey Council. Canadian Bee Industry Safety Quality Traceability Producer Manual: Good Production Practices. 2014. Available at: http://honeycouncil.ca/wp-content/uploads/2016/04/CBISQT-PRODUCER-MANUAL-ver-1.0-16-July-2014-FINAL-distribution-copy-CFIA-approved.pdf. Accessed May 8, 2021.
26. Vidal-Naquet N. Honey bee veterinary medicine: *Apis mellifera L.* Sheffield, United Kingdom: 5m Publishing; 2015.
27. Sebestyen T. Beekeeping basics: seeking her majesty. Am Bee J 2019;159(6): 637–9.
28. Canadian beekeepers' practical Handbook to Bee biosecurity and food safety. 2nd edition. Canada: Canadian Honey Council; 2017. Available at: https://honeycouncil.ca/canadian-beekeepers-practical-handbook-to-bee-biosecurity-and-food-safety/.
29. Dobbelaere W, De Graaf DC, Reybroeck W, et al. Disinfection of wooden structures contaminated with *Paenibacillus larvae* subsp. *larvae* spores. J Appl Microbiol 2001;91(2):212–6.
30. Locke B, Low M, Forsgren E. An integrated management strategy to prevent outbreaks and eliminate infection pressure of American foulbrood disease in a commercial beekeeping operation. Prev Vet Med 2019;167:48–52.
31. Berry JA, Delaplane KS. Effects of comb age on honey bee colony growth and brood survivorship. J Apicultural Res 2001;40(1):3–8.
32. López-Uribe M, Underwood R. Honey bee diseases: American foulbrood. Penn State Extension 2019. Available at: https://extension.psu.edu/honey-bee-diseases-american-foulbrood. Accessed January 10, 2021.
33. Teixeira EW, Guimarães-Cestaro L, Alves MLTMF, et al. Spores of *Paenibacillus larvae, Ascosphaera apis, Nosema ceranae* and *Nosema apis* in bee products supervised by the Brazilian Federal Inspection Service. Rev Brasil Entomol 2018;62(3):188–94.
34. Canadian Food Inspection Agency. National Bee Farm-Level Biosecurity Standard. Government of Canada. 2013. Available at: https://www.inspection.gc.ca/animal-health/terrestrial-animals/biosecurity/standards-and-principles/bee-industry/eng/1365794112591/1365794221593?chap=1. Accessed January 10, 2021.
35. Canadian Food Inspection Agency. Honey Bee Producer Guide to the National Bee Farm-level Biosecurity Standard Appendix E: Honey Bee Biosecurity: Self-Evaluation Checklist. Government of Canada. 2013. Available at: https://www.inspection.gc.ca/animal-health/terrestrial-animals/biosecurity/standards-and-principles/honey-bee-producer-guide/eng/1378390483360/1378390541968?chap=10. Accessed January 10, 2021.

Honeybee (*Apis mellifera*) Health Considerations in Commercial Beekeeping

Daniel Wyns, BS

KEYWORDS

- Commercial beekeeping • Colony transport • Indoor wintering • Shipping bees
- Queen banking

KEY POINTS

- Honeybees kept as livestock in commercial operations can be subject to additional stressors when compared with bees kept at smaller scale or as a hobby.
- Most commercial beekeeping operations are migratory; therefore, good staging, loading, and hauling practices are critical to minimize colony stress.
- Providing colonies for almond pollination in the central valley of California during February and March is an economic driver of the industry that influences year round colony management practices throughout the United States.
- The increasing use of indoor wintering facilities for storage of colonies in controlled conditions before almond pollination is a developing trend within commercial beekeeping that shows promising results for colony health and survival.

INTRODUCTION

Commercial beekeeping operations manage large numbers of honeybee colonies, ranging from a few hundred to tens of thousands. In addition to producing hive products like honey and wax, many operations also produce live bees for sale, such as queens, queen cells, package colonies, nucleus colonies, or full colonies. They also rent out colonies for pollination of a wide variety of crops. Most large-scale operations rely on a blend of revenue from these multiple sources. Often the optimal blend of revenue for an operation is determined by the location or locations of the operation, as the climate and floral resources of the environment largely determine which avenues can be pursued profitably.

Honeybee colonies kept in a commercial context are subject to an array of stressors mentioned throughout this publication but may also face additional stressors that would be absent or decreased outside of the commercial environment. Modern commercial beekeeping almost always involves crop pollination in addition to honey production, and the demands placed on colonies and beekeeping operations by

Michigan State University, 4090 North College Road, Building 0470E, Lansing, MI 48910, USA
E-mail address: Wyns@MSU.edu

Vet Clin Food Anim 37 (2021) 491–503
https://doi.org/10.1016/j.cvfa.2021.06.014
vetfood.theclinics.com

pollination work lead to many management practices and challenges to colony health that are unique to the commercial environment.

COLONY TRANSPORT

Colony transport is an integral part of modern commercial practices, as colonies are frequently moved in order to fulfill pollination contracts, provide access to favorable forage, or seek milder climatic conditions during the winter months. These movements can often span the entire country, and it is not uncommon for large US operations to maintain bases in both a southern and a northern location. Nearly all commercial operations provide colonies for the almond pollination event that occurs throughout the central valley of California during February and March every year (**Fig. 1**). As planted almond acreage grows, the number of colonies required for pollination has been steadily increasing with the estimated 2.5 million colonies required for 2021 almond pollination representing approximately 88% of the colonies in the United States.[1] The income collected from this pollination event is a major contributor to the economic viability of most beekeeping operations. The need to provide an abundance of strong colonies this early in the season has led to many new and evolving management strategies, as many beekeepers manage colonies throughout the year with a primary objective of providing pollination units to almonds. This geography leads to many different migration routes by beekeepers, but it is not at all uncommon to see colonies spend a couple winter months (November to January) in the south, early spring in California almonds (February to March), return to the south for a month (April) or more after almond pollination, and then go to a northern location for further pollination and honey production (May to October).

The aggregation of many of the nation's commercial honeybee "herds" in California provides an opportunity for accelerated disease and parasite transmission because of so many colonies being densely packed into the central valley. When these colonies disperse back across the country, there is potential for any acquired pathogens to be spread rapidly, including elevated risks for stationary colonies that are in proximity to returning migratory colonies.

Because moving colonies is such a prominent part of commercial beekeeping, many commercial operations are palletized. Most commonly, 4 (see **Fig. 1**) or 6 (**Fig. 2**) hives occupy a single pallet to facilitate loading and unloading with forklifts,

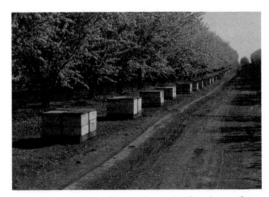

Fig. 1. Nearly a hundred colonies have been placed in this drop of 4-way pallets along an access road to provide pollination for a large almond orchard near Kerman, California. (*Courtesy of* Dan Wyns.)

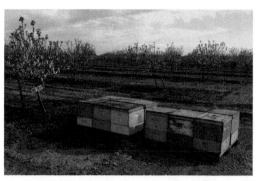

Fig. 2. A dozen colonies on two 6-way pallets are placed at a grower designated "bee drop" location to pollinate a young almond orchard near Lost Hills, California. (*Courtesy of* Dan Wyns.)

skid steers, or occasionally boom loaders. Short moves are typically undertaken with light- and medium-duty flat deck trucks during periods of cold or dark when bees are not flying (**Fig. 3**). Moving colonies relatively short distances during a time of no-flight activity can be accomplished without wrapping the loaded hives under nets. Longer moves like coming and going from California or to/from wintering locations is typically accomplished with semitrucks (**Fig. 4**). Because these long-distance hauls often occur over multiple days with some daylight travel and variable temperatures en route, the loads are netted to confine bees while still allowing airflow to minimize colony stress (**Fig. 5**). When planning and discussing large-scale migratory matters, commercial beekeepers often speak in terms of loads, referencing a full semitrailer full of bees. The number of hives in a load can vary depending on hive size and pallet dimensions, with 408 and 432 being common quantities for loads of full-size hives, but smaller hives may allow for more hives per load. The number of hives per load is a function of both space and weight. The hauling of bees has become a specialized skill within the trucking industry with continual improvements being sought.

Honeybee colonies generate a large amount of heat, and in general, it is important that loads of bees do not sit idle without the ventilation provided by movement for long periods of times, particularly in direct sunlight or hot temperatures. Many experienced bee haulers know of locations along their common routes where they can stop to refuel or rest while minimizing stress to the bees or potential for public nuisance.

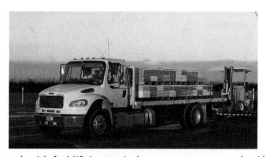

Fig. 3. A flat deck truck with forklift in tow is the most common method beekeepers use for short-distance loading and hauling. (*Courtesy of* Dan Wyns.)

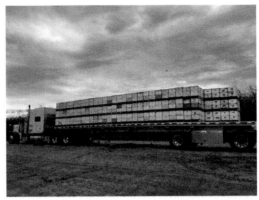

Fig. 4. A load of hives ready to be unloaded into a holding yard after transport. (*Courtesy of* Matt Hoepfinger.)

Inspection Stations

Interstate transport of bees typically requires a health certificate, although requirements vary among states. Health inspections are carried out by state apiarists (or a qualified authority in a similar position) in the location from which the colonies are departing and must be provided in the destination state when required. Inspection procedures and authorized personnel vary between states. More information on inspections for interstate transportation is available from the Apiary Inspectors of America.[2] In addition to health certificates for the bees, loads crossing state lines may be required to stop for inspections to verify they are free of certain potentially invasive organisms (ants, weed seeds, and so forth). These inspections are carried out at dedicated agricultural inspection stations at state entry points and are especially common for loads entering California. Delays at these inspection stations can cause stress to colonies, particularly during hot weather conditions. Some of the inspection stations have water sources available so that loads may be hosed down for cooling purposes while they are waiting to pass through.[3]

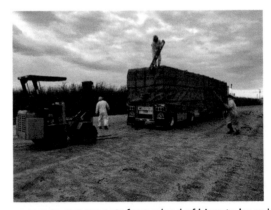

Fig. 5. Beekeepers prepare to remove nets from a load of hives to be unloaded into a holding yard before almond bloom. (*Courtesy of* Photo Matt Hoepfinger.)

Bee Truck Crashes

With the abundance of bees being transported nationwide, it is inevitable that accidents occur. Accidents involving bee trucks, although rare, do happen with often devastating results. First responders are often not equipped or prepared to respond as they typically would to an accident when the accident scene includes millions of stinging bees. When incidents occur, it is common for calls to go out to the local beekeeping community for experienced beekeepers in the area to render assistance. First responders are often limited to controlling traffic from a safe distance until the potential for mass stinging can be reduced. Often in bee truck accidents, much of the hive woodware is heavily damaged. The resulting chaos often takes time for the bees to settle and beekeepers to make judgments on how many of the colonies are salvageable. Normally much of the load cannot be saved, and equipment may be doused with foam to control and euthanize displaced bees before damaged equipment can be sorted through and removed.

Prolonged Season

The migratory nature of commercial beekeeping, particularly the reliance of many operations on the income provided by almond pollination during February in California, has led to colonies having a much longer active season with a relatively short (if at all) period of dormancy in the winter. With colonies needing to be strong in February to make grade for almond contracts, they are often stimulated to reduce or bypass winter dormancy. The increased period whereby brood is present in the colonies, year-round in some operations, means that varroa mites can reproduce for an extended duration or the entire year. The early stimulation to colonies provided by resources foraged and supplied before and during almond pollination leads to larger colonies earlier in the year but also leads to increased varroa mite reproduction. Although this early start to varroa mite growth may not be immediately detrimental to colony health, it can become problematic later in the season. The exponential growth of varroa populations means an extra generation or 2 can lead to significantly higher infestation levels later in the season.

COMMERCIAL APIARIES

Commercial apiaries vary in number of colonies depending on the purpose of the yard and abundance of forage in the surrounding landscape (**Fig. 6**). In determining apiary size, there is a balance to be struck between the efficiency of maintaining large numbers of colonies in a single location against the amount of forage (carrying capacity) of a location and potential for increased disease pressure in larger aggregations of colonies.

Drift and Robbing

Aggregating a large number of colonies in a single apiary increases the interaction between colonies and potential for pathogen transmission. This interaction between colonies can occur via drift and robbing. Drift is the term beekeepers use to describe individual bees from one colony returning to another colony after a foraging flight. Honeybee foragers are very good at navigating for several miles across the landscape, but when returning to an apiary site containing dozens of hives often painted to look identical, some of these foragers will end up in different hives. As these foragers return with resources for the colony, they are not barred from entry by the guard bees as is often the case for robber bees. It has been shown that the increased drift within crowded apiaries can result in colonies being more vulnerable to damage from varroa mites

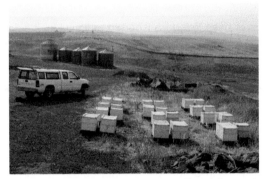

Fig. 6. Commercial apiaries, like this one near Grangeville, Idaho, typically contain dozens of palletized colonies in a compact space and, are often located within the margins of the agricultural landscape. (*Courtesy of* Dan Wyns.)

and the viruses they carry.[4] Jay[5,6] provides an overview of the environmental factors and hive placements within commercial apiaries that influence the degree to which drift occurs.

Whereas drift can be considered a passive way in which bees from one colony interact with another, robbing is a behavior whereby foragers from one colony deliberately seek out small or weak colonies from which they can steal honey (**Fig. 7**). Although robbing is not unique to colonies in a commercial setting, the larger apiary size can mean more potential robbers in immediate proximity. In commercial apiaries with high colony numbers, there may be reduced time available for a beekeeper to

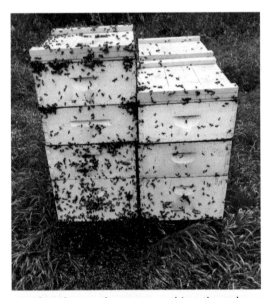

Fig. 7. Robbing events where bees seek entrance to hives through any gap or crack in an effort to steal honey can be particularly problematic in large commercial apiaries and highlight the importance of maintaining good-quality woodware that is bee-tight and working through necessary in hive tasks quickly. (*Courtesy of* Ana Heck.)

perform necessary tasks in an apiary before a robbing frenzy has been initiated and escalates to damaging levels. Robbing is not limited to within a single apiary, as bees will potentially cover an area of several miles in search of an opportunity to steal honey. Robbing is particularly common and problematic in the late summer and fall when colony populations remain high and many locations see nectar dearth conditions following the main period of honey flow.

Robbing is difficult to curtail once started; therefore, prevention as much as possible is advised. Generally maintaining clean beekeeping practices like avoiding discarding comb scrapings or spillage during feeding can reduce or delay the onset of robbing. It is also advisable to not open hives for longer than necessary during times of the season when robbing activity is common.

Holding/Loading Yards

Because moving bees is an integral part of most commercial beekeeping operations, many outfits maintain several sites specifically suited to aggregating large numbers of colonies for brief periods of loading and unloading trucks (**Fig. 8**). These yards are typically called loading or holding yards. Before loading a semitruck for long-distance moves, colonies from the surrounding production apiaries or pollination locations are brought into a holding yard in the nights before loading trucks. When hauled in from the surrounding area, the colonies are typically stacked 2 or 3 pallets high on the trucks used to transport colonies to the holding yard (**Fig. 9**). Often these stacked pallets are removed from trucks and remain in their stacks for several days until they are loaded onto semitrucks for long-distance travel (**Fig. 10**). This practice of leaving colonies stacked can lead to increased drift between colonies, but this drift is traded for the time saved unstacking and restacking the columns between unloading and loading. The aggregation process is often repeated at the other end of the journey, with beekeepers unloading semitrucks at a central holding yard and then distributing hives to pollination contracts or honey production sites with smaller trucks over subsequent nights.

INDOOR WINTERING STORAGE

The wintering period is a time when a colony of honeybees enters a state of dormancy. Although not a true hibernation, the dormancy involves reduced activity with infrequent exiting of the hive. Brood rearing during this period also slows or stops. During

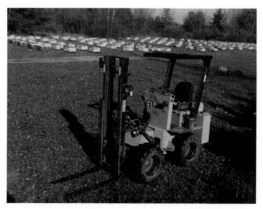

Fig. 8. A forklift is used to stack and load the hives in this holding yard for transport. (*Courtesy of* Dan Wyns.)

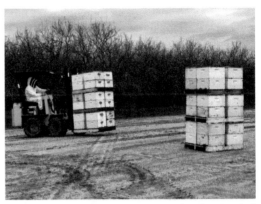

Fig. 9. Stacked pallets provide more efficient loading and unloading in holding yards before dispersal for pollination contracts. (*Courtesy of* Matt Hoepfinger.)

periods of cold weather, the bees in the hive cluster together to thermoregulate. Bees vibrate their flight muscles to generate heat to keep the cluster temperature constant. The colony relies on the honey stores gathered earlier in the year to provide the necessary calories.

Bee activity and cluster density are directly influenced by ambient temperature. Warmer temperatures increase activity, and the cluster loosens; if it is sufficiently warm, some bees may briefly exit the hive for a cleansing flight. Bees in a clustered colony are metabolically most efficient at an ambient temperature near 40°F (about 4.5°C).[7] Increased bee activity brought on by higher temperatures leads to greater honey consumption. Bees also consume more honey in order to generate adequate heat for the cluster, as temperatures get much lower. Daily temperature fluctuations during the winter can result in increased consumption of honey stores, and therefore, maintaining a constant ambient temperature will allow the colony to minimize consumption of honey. To this end, commercial beekeepers are increasingly using indoor storage facilities where temperature can be controlled in order to provide optimal conditions for winter dormancy.

Indoor wintering continues to increase in popularity, particularly among commercial beekeepers seeking to provide colonies for almond pollination shortly after they

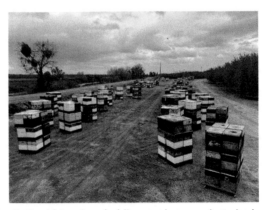

Fig. 10. Stacks of palletized hives in a holding yard are ready to be loaded for transport. (*Courtesy of* Matt Hoepfinger.)

emerge from storage. Storing colonies in controlled conditions results in more predictable outcomes as far as colony size, health, and consumption of honey stores than colonies that winter in more variable environmental conditions. This more predictable outcome is valuable to beekeepers, as it is economically important to be able to forecast the number and size of colonies they can expect to send to pollination.

Early US adopters of indoor wintering were beekeepers who used potato storage facilities that were not in use during the winter months. The partially subterranean shelters were designed to reduce temperature fluctuations by using the thermal mass of the surrounding ground while also having exhaust systems capable of moving enough volume of air. The success of these early experiences wintering bees in structures led beekeepers to construct facilities for the purpose of wintering. McCutcheon[8] provides a detailed history of the adoption and early advances in indoor wintering experiences in Canada and the United States.

Honeybee colonies generate a tremendous amount of heat, and large aggregations of stored colonies require a facility that can be kept within the optimal storage temperature range of 37°F to 42°F (2.8°C–5.6°C) and that can also maintain other appropriate atmospheric conditions.[9] This cooling is most often accomplished by continually drawing cold external air into the facility and venting exhaust. Some facilities are insulated and refrigerated to provide active cooling capacity, especially in warmer locations. Indoor wintering facilities may also have misting systems built into the ceiling. These misting capabilities provide a measure of emergency cooling when external temperatures are too high to keep colonies cool enough with air exchange alone.

Air flow in a storage facility is important, and colonies are organized and stacked accordingly. Pallets of colonies are stacked in columns, often up to 6 pallets high. Parallel rows of these stacks should be placed so that there is space between rows, allowing dead bees on the ground to be swept periodically. Within a row of stacks, each stack should be separated from adjacent stacks by a few inches. This small space is important, as it discourages bees that emerge from hives from entering a neighboring hive as they could if adjacent pallets were touching. Bees will not fly in the dark conditions of a wintering facility. Red lights may be used to allow human visibility within the facility without causing the bees to become active and fly.

In 2020, Project Apis m., in collaboration with researchers and industry stakeholders, developed an excellent resource that provides detailed coverage of the most current best practices and scientific advances in relation to indoor wintering of colonies. The guide, entitled *Indoor Storage of Honey Bee Colonies in the US*, is available for PDF download[9] at: https://www.projectapism.org/indoor-storage-guide-for-honey-bees.html.

SHIPPING PACKAGE COLONIES AND QUEENS

As discussed above, the movement of honeybee colonies of various sizes is an integral part of most commercial beekeeping operations. Colonies being moved can vary in size, but a hive typically contains a population of bees, including a queen, as well as the combs with brood and food stores contained within. Although these colonies are considered to be "bees on comb," there is another subset of bee transport that involves bees, not on comb, but rather specially packaged in temporary containers for transport. The 2 most common ways that bees are shipped without comb is either as package colonies or queens.

A package colony of bees, often simply referred to as a package, consists of a defined weight of adult bees (3 lb, about 1.3 kg, is common) with a mated queen enclosed in a queen cage, as well as a container of syrup or food, all contained within a box designed to provide ventilation during transport while still containing the included bees. Loads of packages are most commonly transported via truck (**Fig. 11**), although international shipments may travel by air cargo. Packages in transport should not be subjected to prolonged periods of direct sunlight or temperature extremes, as their ability to adequately thermoregulate may be overwhelmed.

Beekeepers have developed shipping methods and packaging to minimize stress to bees during transport. Queens are shipped in individual cages (**Fig. 12**) that are placed in racks designed to hold each queen cage securely with mesh surfaces oriented to allow ventilation and access by attendant worker bees. The rack or racks of caged queens are secured inside of a cardboard shipping box (**Fig. 13**) with ventilation on opposing sides to promote airflow. Shipping boxes are specifically designed for the bee industry and are most commonly referred to as battery boxes. Once the racks of queens are secured in the battery box, a source of food (fondant) and water (damp sponge) is also affixed inside the box. After provisioning the battery box, it is supplied with bulk bees to act as attendants during transport. These attendants will provide the queens with food and water during transport and work collectively to thermoregulate. It is important that the battery box be supplied with enough attendants to keep the queens warm, including those at the perimeter when cooler temperatures cause clustering.

Battery boxes come in different sizes and are labeled to indicate that they contain live bees and that they should not be left in direct sunlight. Excessively high temperatures during transport can overcome the attendants' ability to ventilate adequately and lead to thermal damage. Prolonged or extreme heat can be lethal to shipped queens, but sublethal damage that is not readily apparent is also possible.

Because of the value and relative fragility of a battery box full of queens, they are frequently shipped using next-day or 2-day airmail. Beekeepers who frequently ship or receive queens will often work with their postal carrier or local courier to communicate best handling practices during transit. It is often possible to request notification when the bees arrive at local shipping hubs where they can be directly retrieved by the beekeeper rather than have them exposed to the extended duration and variable conditions of time on a local delivery truck.

BANKING QUEENS

Within the commercial beekeeping realm, there are many producers who specialize in breeding and rearing large numbers of queens to supply other beekeepers. Many operations that run colonies for pollination or honey production purchase large quantities of queens from these specialty producers in order to requeen existing colonies or

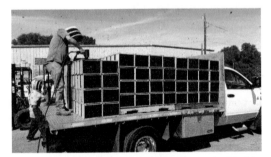

Fig. 11. A load of several hundred honeybee packages in mesh-sided boxes are stacked and secured by the beekeeper to ensure good ventilation during transport. (*Courtesy of* Ben Sallman.)

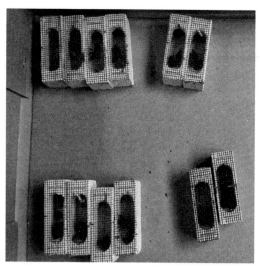

Fig. 12. Queens are confined to individual queen cages before being secured in a battery box with attendant bees for shipment. (*Courtesy of* Ben Sallman.)

make new units by splitting colonies. The ability to divide a colony into multiple units by dividing bees, brood, and colony resources and then adding purchased queens where needed is a significant part of many beekeeping operations. Splitting colonies allows beekeepers to grow colony numbers, replace dead colonies, or sell splits or full-sized colonies. Queen rearing and use of these queens require a great deal of planning to receive queens when needed and have colonies ready and waiting to receive them, but even with careful scheduling, many situations arise where queens need to be stored for a period of time before installation. This storing of queens is referred to as banking.

Queen banking involves artificially manipulating a colony so that many caged, mated queens can be stored there for an extended period of time. When correctly executed, queen banking creates a situation whereby the host colony (queen bank) provides the thermoregulation for the individual queens as well as feeding and attending to the banked queens. There are multiple methods for establishing and

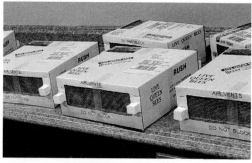

Fig. 13. Battery boxes each contain up to a hundred queens in individual cages and are provisioned with fondant, water, and attendant bees to care for the queens and thermoregulate during transit. (*Courtesy of* Ben Sallman.)

maintaining a queen bank. The best method will depend on the number of queens to be banked and the duration of intended storage. Each individual queen to be stored in a bank needs to be in her own individual queen cage.

Queens can be banked for a short period inside of a well-ventilated battery (shipping) box that is kept away from extreme temperatures and out of direct sunlight. Battery box queen banks are often taken into the field by beekeepers to have queens available when making splits or requeening colonies.

When banking queens in an actual hive, a colony that has been made intentionally queenless is used. There should be plenty of young bees present in the bank, and it may be beneficial to shake extra young bees from another colony to supplement the population. If the bank is to be maintained for an extended period, the population should be maintained by regularly adding frames of capped, ready to emerge, brood or periodically shaking in additional young bees from another queenright colony. The beekeeper may need to periodically check for and cull queen cells from added brood frames in the queen bank so that a queen does not emerge. Queen banks should be well fed with syrup and protein if not naturally abundant. Several hundred queens can be stored in a single bank, although a lower density is recommended as the limited ability of nurse bees to care for that many queens may lead to suboptimal care. Queen cages should be arranged in the bank so that a screened portion of every queen cage is accessible to the nurse bees in the colony. Specially modified banking frames are available that hold queen cages with the mesh exposed to provide easy access by the nurse bees. When banking queens, it is critical that every cage have a secure plug that cannot be chewed by bees. Fondant or other chewable substances that may plug holes in queen cages can result in queens being inadvertently released from their cages.

CLINICS CARE POINTS

- Commercial beekeepers typically make colony management decisions regarding feeding, medication, and treatments at the apiary or operational level rather than individual colony level.
- It is common for one or multiple beekeeping tasks (feeding, requeening, medicating, harvesting honey, and so forth) to be performed on all colonies within the operation over the course of a week or multiple weeks, and then all the colonies are cycled through again with this pattern repeated throughout the year for each management action.
- Problems within an operation (eg, high varroa mite pressure) may be recognized but difficult to address in a timely manner because of the number of colonies under management and geographic distribution; therefore, proactive monitoring and preventive actions are to be encouraged.
- Veterinarians working with commercial beekeepers should understand that decisions regarding colony management and health are made in the context of the financial considerations, including cost of inputs (including labor) and expected outcomes.
- Veterinarians with migratory beekeeper clients should work with the client to proactively develop a plan of action should the client require veterinary services when hives are located outside of the state in which the veterinarian is licensed.

DISCLOSURE

The author has no commercial or financial conflicts of interest related to this document.

REFERENCES

1. Goodrich BK, Durant JL. 2021 Almond pollination outlook: economic outlook and other considerations. Fresno, CA: West Coast Nut; 2020. p. 12–8. Available at: https://www.wcngg.com/2020/11/23/2021-almond-pollination-outlook-economic-outlook-and-other-considerations/. Accessed December 22, 2020.
2. Apiary inspectors of America. Available at: https://apiaryinspectors.org/us-inspection-services/. Accessed December 22, 2020.
3. California Department of Food and Agriculture. Available at: https://www.cdfa.ca.gov/plant/pollinators/inspections.html. Accessed January 3, 2021.
4. Seeley TD, Smith ML. Crowding honeybee colonies in apiaries can increase their vulnerability to the deadly ectoparasite *Varroa destructor*. Apidologie 2015;46: 716–27.
5. Jay SC. Drifting of honeybees in commercial apiaries I: effect of various environmental factors. J Apic Res 1965;4(3):167–75.
6. Jay SC. Drifting of honeybees in commercial apiaries. III: effect of apiary layout. J Apic Res 1966;5(3):137–48.
7. Southwick EE. Metabolic energy of intact honey bee colonies. Comp Biochem Physiol A Physiol 1982;71(2):277–81.
8. McCutcheon DM. Indoor wintering of hives. Bee World 1984;65(1):19–37.
9. Hopkins BK, editor. Indoor storage of honey bee colonies in the United States. 2020. Available at: https://www.projectapism.org/indoor-storage-guide-for-honey-bees.html. Accessed January 6, 2021.

Honey Bee Nutrition

Jennifer M. Tsuruda, PhD[a], Priyadarshini Chakrabarti, PhD[b,c],
Ramesh R. Sagili, PhD[c],*

KEYWORDS

- Honey bee nutrition • Foraging behavior • Supplemental forage
- Nutritional supplements

KEY POINTS

- Honey bee nutrition is complex and unique, and is not analogous to that of other livestock/animals.
- Pollen (protein) and nectar (carbohydrate) are the primary food resources collected by honey bees.
- Foraging behavior of honey bees depends on both inside colony environment and external environment.
- Beekeepers provide supplemental nutrition (protein and sugars) to their colonies during foraging dearths.

 Video content accompanies this article at http://www.vetfood.theclinics.com.

CHALLENGES ASSOCIATED WITH HONEY BEE NUTRITION

Honey bee nutrition is complex and unique and is not analogous to that of other livestock/animals, where nutritional needs of specific animals are well understood and appropriate diets/feed have been formulated. Honey bees are social insects, and the colony is considered a superorganism with a well-defined caste system and reproductive division of labor. Similar to their complex biology, nutrition is also complex in honey bees and can be considered at 3 levels (1) colony nutrition, (2) adult nutrition, and (3) larval nutrition.[1] As they age, honey bee workers transition from high-essential-amino-acid diets to predominantly carbohydrate diets.[2]

Honey bee nutrition is highly dependent on the environment, that is, the floral composition of the landscape.[3] Honey bees encounter dynamically changing floral resources in the landscape, in both space and time.[4] The quantity and quality of these floral resources are also dynamic throughout the year.[5] Hence, honey bees

J.M. Tsuruda and P. Chakrabarti contributed equally to this work.
[a] University of Tennessee - Knoxville, 2505 E J Chapman Drive, Knoxville, TN 37996, USA;
[b] Mississippi State University, P.O. Box 5307, Mississippi State, MS 39762, USA; [c] Oregon State University, 4017 Agriculture and Life Science Building, Corvallis, OR 97331, USA
* Corresponding author.
E-mail address: ramesh.sagili@oregonstate.edu

Vet Clin Food Anim 37 (2021) 505–519
https://doi.org/10.1016/j.cvfa.2021.06.006
0749-0720/21/© 2021 The Authors. Published by Elsevier Inc.

may face significant challenges in terms of pollen diversity, quantity, and quality based on their geographic location. At present, efforts are underway across the country to improve nutrition for diversity of bees (including managed bees such as honey bees and wild bees such as many native bee species) by planting forage. A major limitation of this approach is that the target forage species are chosen predominantly based on their apparent attractiveness to bees and not based on the nutritional composition of pollen and nectar or the nutritional needs of the bees. However, beekeepers have access to supplements that exclusively provide protein but do not provide other required essential nutrients. Furthermore, there are huge gaps in knowledge regarding honey bee nutrition, and hence, to date, no optimal/balanced diet is available for honey bees.

FORAGING BEHAVIOR OF HONEY BEES

Foraging behavior reflects the interdependence between pollinators and plants and involves several factors from within the hive as well as from the outside environment. Diversity of available floral resources (or lack thereof) across a foraging range or across time and seasons can result in different levels and types of behavior and collected resources, which can have cascading effects on the colony's growth, survival, and reproduction.

Factors Influencing Foraging Behavior

There are several biological factors, including the genetics and physiology of honey bees, underlying foraging behavior outside of the nutritional quality of resources. The amount of brood (developing larvae) and the levels of brood pheromone affect foraging behaviors. The larvae depend on a diet made from collected pollen, although the response may be threshold based and foragers can also revert back to nursing behavior if there are insufficient numbers of nurse bees to tend to the amount of larvae.[6-9] High levels of stored pollen can cause a negative feedback effect that inhibits pollen foraging by recruiting fewer numbers of pollen foragers, fewer trips to collect pollen, and/or smaller amounts of pollen collected during a trip.[6,10,11] Genetic variation also underlies differential foraging behavior and responses to foraging stimuli, as revealed by the selection for bees that collect and hoard high and low amounts of pollen, and the identification of regions of the genome and candidate genes associated with foraging age (the age at which young workers initiate foraging) and specialization (pollen vs nectar).[12,13] In addition, the reproductive physiology of a functionally sterile worker can influence foraging age and specialization.[14-16]

There are also factors outside of the hive that influence a bee's foraging choices. Bumble bees have been shown to forage on pollens according to their nutritional values, whereas honey bee studies have had mixed results, with some showing bees choosing to forage on and dance for pollen resources of lower quality.[17-21] However, honey bee colonies have a complex social structure, with the superorganism having a common, centralized "stomach." Foraging efforts may be adjusted in response to multiple factors to achieve overall optimal nutrition.[22]

Foraging Range and Recruitment

The nutritional needs of a colony change across a year as do the availability of resources, which impacts the growth of a colony. However, bees can adjust their foraging efforts and range to seek out new food patches. Relative to most other bees, honey bees have a wide foraging range with von Frisch[23] reporting the foraging range to be up to 13.5 km. Although many studies have reported foraging distances between 0.7 and 2.0 km, wider ranges have also been reported and have been shown to vary by month and forage type.[24,25]

Foraging efficiency is a determinant of foraging distances, and energy spent by individual bees is balanced with gains to the colony.[26,27] Flight is an energetically expensive activity, needing thoracic flight muscles to be greater than a minimum of around 30°C.[28,29] Environmental factors (eg, air temperature and solar radiation) can affect body temperature, but in general, the longer the distances traveled to resources, the lower the efficiency and higher the likelihood of needing to fuel their flights with more sugar for meeting the higher energy demands.[27,28,30]

The communication and recruitment behavior of honey bees has long fascinated researchers and nonscientists. von Frisch[23] documented and described the waggle dance, a figure-eight movement of returning foragers that involves vibration of the abdomen while moving in a linear line (Video 1). The length of the dance and the angle/orientation of the vibratory movement reflect the distance and direction of resources relative to the sun.[23] Other bees observing the dance may be recruited to forage at the same location. This behavior continues to be studied in several contexts, including foraging preference, pollen diversity, communication, and conflict.[31–33] Odors, colors, and memory also provide context to foraging and recruitment.[34,35]

NUTRITIONAL NEEDS OF HONEY BEES

Honey bees are often called superorganisms[36] because of their social structure. In addition to an absence of diseases, a healthy colony must be able to sustain functioning members (workers and reproductives) capable of performing their tasks and resisting various abiotic and biotic stressors.[1]

Consuming sufficient quantities of high-quality pollen (**Fig. 1**) has been shown to decrease susceptibility to the gut parasite *Nosema ceranae*, lower pathogen loads, improve honey bee immunity and overwintering success, improve semen quality in drones, and result in healthier honey bees that are better able to counteract pesticide stress, disease incidences, transportation stress, and parasitic pressures.[1,37–41] Other

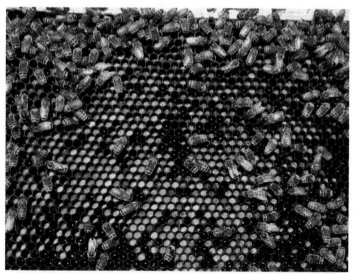

Fig. 1. A frame of pollen from multiple plant sources as evident from the different colors.

studies have associated nutrition with bee behavior. The physiology of the emergent spring workers may be affected by nutrition, which subsequently may alter their behavior.[42] Larvae with restricted access to optimal nutrition developed into inefficient foraging and waggle-dancing adults.[43] The ratio of pollen protein:lipid may also guide the foraging preferences in bee pollinators.[44] Thus, optimal nutrition may be considered as the honey bee colony's first line of defense, enabling it to better withstand both biotic and abiotic stress.

As with the nutritional requirements for other animals, bee nutrients can be largely classified as macronutrients and micronutrients. As the name suggests, macronutrients are required in large quantities and are critical for the development and sustenance of honey bees. Examples include proteins, carbohydrates, and lipids. Micronutrients are equally important, even though they are required in smaller quantities. Vitamins, minerals, phytochemicals, and phytosterols are examples of the micronutrients required by honey bees. Carbohydrate-rich nectar is the primary energy source for bees and contains important phytochemicals, whereas pollen provides vital proteins, lipids, vitamins, phytosterols, and phytochemicals.[1,38,45] In polymorphic eusocial insect societies, such as in honey bee colonies, developmental nutritional conditions shape caste determination.[46] Thus, for a healthy honey bee colony to thrive, an optimal balance of all macronutrients and micronutrients is needed.

Macronutrients

Carbohydrates

Nectar and honey dew (sugar-rich liquid, secreted by some insects, such as aphids, when they feed on plant sap) are the natural sources of carbohydrates for honey bees. Foragers collect nectar and honey dew from plants and store it in their crops (honey stomachs) for transportation back to the hive. Then it is gradually converted to honey in the colony by the addition of invertase and other enzymes[47] and the reduction of water.[48] Honey is stored in cells for feeding the colony[1] and is an important staple for brood rearing and overwintering.

Compared with larvae, adult honey bees have low glycogen stores.[49] The differences in carbohydrate use between the adult honey bees and the larvae may be attributed to the differences in metabolic enzymes.[50] A worker bee needs about 11 mg dry sugar per day, and a colony with 50,000 bees needs approximately 700 lb (~318 kg) sugar per year.[51] As most floral nectars contain less than 50% sugar, the amount of nectar needed to support a large colony and its carbohydrate needs are thus much higher than 700 lb (~318 kg) (of nectar) annually.[51]

Proteins

Pollen is the primary source of protein in a honey bee colony. The protein content of pollen ranges from 2.5% to 61%.[52] Ten amino acids in specific proportions are essential for honey bees and must be acquired through diets: arginine, histidine, isoleucine, leucine, lysine, methionine, phenylalanine, threonine, tryptophan, and valine.[53] These amino acids are essential for reproduction, growth, and development.[50] Some examples of good pollen sources, even though having short blooming periods, include sweet clovers, mustards, and rapeseed.[54,55]

A colony having 20,000 honey bees collects about 125 lb (~57 kg) of pollen annually, and approximately 15% to 30% of the foragers are pollen foragers in a colony.[56] The workers further process the collected pollen that has been brought back to the hive and store it as "bee bread." The total pollen consumptions by nurse bees within a short span of 10 days is approximately 65 mg per bee after which the consumption of pollen decreases.[57] Nurse bees biosynthesize proteinaceous secretions in their hypopharyngeal glands by consuming pollens, which are then progressively provisioned to the developing larvae and referred to as brood food.[57,58] The worker-destined larvae are fed worker jelly (protein-rich secretions for the first 2 days and then a mixture of protein secretions, pollen, and nectar for the next 3 days) by nurse bees, and the queen-destined larvae are fed royal jelly exclusively throughout their development.[59-61]

For rearing a single larva, 25 to 37.5 mg protein is required, which is comparable to 125 to 187.5 mg pollen.[49] A shortage in pollen therefore not only may decrease the number of individuals within the honey bee colony[62] but also may result in increased susceptibility to other stressors.[37,63,64]

Lipids
Lipids in pollen range from 1% to 20% by weight,[52] of which essential fatty acids are a crucial component. Essential fatty acids such as linoleic and γ-linoleic acids comprise 0.4% and phospholipids comprise 1.5%[65,66] of the total lipid fraction. Apart from supporting the essential physiologic functions, fatty acids, such as oleic acid, have been shown to enhance learning and survival in bumble bees.[67] Studies have also shown that low omega 6:omega-3 fatty acid ratios enhance learning performances in honey bees.[68] Based on the lipid preferences of particular bee species (specialists or generalists), the choice of host plants may vary during foraging.[69] Examples of neutral lipids in pollen include glycerides, free fatty acids, sterols, sterol esters, and hydrocarbons.[70] Of these, sterols are a vital micronutrient.

Micronutrients

Phytosterols
Sterols are a form of lipid, playing vital physiologic roles in insects, which include acting as a precursor of important molting hormones and also forming the building blocks of cellular membranes.[71,72] For honey bees, the most vital phytosterol is 24-methylenecholesterol. Studies have shown that caged honey bees fed artificial diets supplemented with 24-methylenecholesterol had longer survival and had more brood production, when compared with honey bees fed a different phytosterol in the artificial diets.[73] This sterol is also the major sterol ($\sim 50\%$) in honey bee pupae.[74] Honey bees are not able to interconvert C28 and C29 phytosterols, and nurse bees are able to progressively assimilate this sterol in their tissues[75] and selectively transfer these sterols through the brood food to the growing larvae.[76,77] Thus, to produce ecdysteroids (makisterone-A) from sterols, honey bees exclusively depend on their diets for 24-methylenecholesterol. Recent studies have also highlighted the important physiologic impacts of 24-methylenecholesterol on honey bees, including increase in bee longevity and enhancement in head protein and abdominal lipid contents.[75,78,79] With evidence showing that plant pollens have a diversity of sterol compositions,[45] it is important that bees have access to diverse flora to source the required phytosterols.

Phytochemicals
Phytochemicals in nectar have largely been considered beneficial for honey bees. Phenolic acids and flavonols are the most common phytochemicals[80] found in nectar other than alkaloids and terpenoids,[81] with compositions and concentrations varying largely depending on the floral taxa.[82] Of the phenolic acids and flavonols, 2 compounds are notable for their immense benefits in improving honey bee health: p-coumaric acid and quercetin. Studies have shown that phytochemical consumptions by honey bees enhance longevity, reduce *Nosema* infection, upregulate honey bee genes with antimicrobial properties, and counteract pesticide stress.[39,80,83,84]

NUTRITIONAL SUPPLEMENTS

Protein

Beekeepers in North America generally provide protein supplements to honey bee colonies during foraging dearth (especially during fall and late fall) and spring to boost colony strength by enhancing brood rearing[42,85] (**Fig. 2**). Also, honey bee colonies used for crop pollination often face nutritional stress because the quality or quantity of pollen forage available to them in such agricultural landscapes can be inadequate.[63] Fall and late fall feeding of protein is critical, because this is the time when winter bees (diutinus) are reared in the colonies and these bees are vital for overwintering survival of colonies. However, current protein supplements available to beekeepers do not sustain long-term brood rearing in honey bee colonies. Some studies have reported that colonies fed protein supplements do not perform as well when compared with colonies receiving real pollen.[40,64,86]

Most of the protein supplements available in the market for honey bees are either whey or soy-based products. Some of these available supplements have a small percentage of pollen added to the protein supplement. Although protein supplements are not equivalent to pollen in terms of nutrient composition, several studies have reported enhanced brood rearing and low disease susceptibility associated with the use of protein supplements.[87–89] The commercial beekeepers in the Pacific Northwest feed on average 1.8 kg protein supplement in spring and about 1.8 to 3.6 kg in fall.[90] Although it is not easy to diagnose nutritional stress in a colony, there are visual symptoms that may indicate severe nutritional stress such as larvae with low or no brood food in their respective cells (**Fig. 3**). The larvae reared in honey bee colonies with ample pollen stores are normally bathed in a sufficient supply of brood food provisioned by nurse bees.

Carbohydrate

Similar to protein, beekeepers also provide sugar to their colonies during times of nectar dearth (especially during fall and late fall periods) and inclement weather.

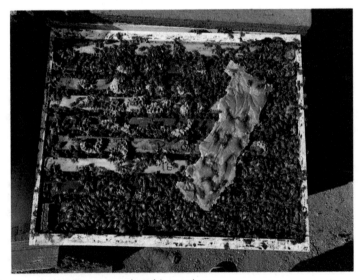

Fig. 2. Protein supplement patty placed in a colony.

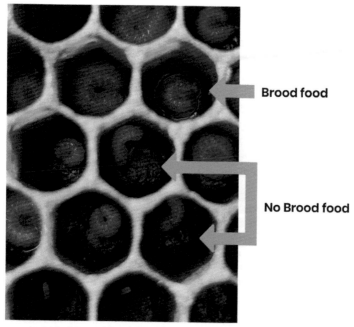

Brood food

No Brood food

Fig. 3. Larvae devoid of brood food (larval starvation symptom).

Honey bee colonies are mostly fed liquid sugar syrup during spring and fall and are provided dry sugar or fondant (**Fig. 4**) during the winter period when bees do not prefer sugar syrup due to lower temperatures. Winter starvation can result when access to stored honey is limited, commonly seen as many inward-facing, dead honey bees in frames (**Fig. 5**); however, inward-facing dead honey bees in frames is not a definitive

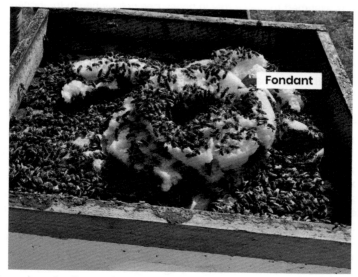

Fondant

Fig. 4. Honey bees feeding on fondant during winter.

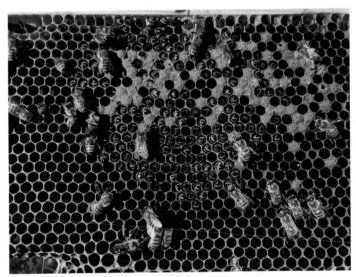

Fig. 5. Dead honey bees facing inward into cells (adult starvation symptom).

diagnosis for starvation. In spring, the concentration of sugar syrup fed to colonies is about 50%, and it is about 66% during fall or late fall. The commercial beekeepers in the Pacific Northwest report feeding their colonies between 5 and 15 L of sugar syrup in spring and 10 and 25 L in the autumn.[90]

Probiotics

Honey bee gut microbiome research is an emerging field.[91] The honey bee worker guts contain a distinctive community of about 8 dominant bacterial species.[92] The gut bacteria may play several important roles in honey bees, including a role in nutrition by assisting in digestion (carbohydrate metabolism).[92,93] Even though the gut microbiota is assumed to play a role in honey bee colony health (pathogen defense) and nutrition, the specific functions of each of these dominant gut bacteria are currently unknown.[94] Over the past 3 years, some beekeepers have started using commercially available probiotics marketed for honey bees. These commercial probiotics claim to improve digestion and support gut health and colony health. Unfortunately, to date, there is a paucity of peer-reviewed published research regarding the benefits of these commercial probiotics to honey bees.

Supplemental Forage and Integrating Floral Diversity into Cropping Systems

Another promising option for improving bee nutrition is providing supplemental forage.[40,95,96] Honey bee colonies with access to supplemental forage have been reported to experience lower mortality when compared with colonies that did not have access to supplemental forage.[97] Over the past few years, there has been a significant emphasis on improving pollinator forage and habitat to boost bee health in the wake of colony declines, including the 2014 Presidential Memorandum for creating a federal strategy to promote the health of honey bees and other pollinators. Some nonprofit agencies such as the Project *Apis m* (https://www.projectapism.org/seeds-for-bees.html) have developed programs like Seeds for Bees that encourage the use of cover crops in orchards and farms to improve forage for bees. Another nonprofit organization called the Xerces Society has developed a comprehensive list of pollinator-friendly plants that are highly attractive to pollinators, including native bees and honey bees (https://xerces.org/pollinator-conservation/pollinator-friendly-plant-lists). At present, pollinator plants chosen for habitat development are based on their apparent attractiveness to bees. There is little information regarding the quality of forage (especially pollen quality) available to bees. A more scientific way to choose these plants should be based on the nutritional composition of their pollens, which vary widely in their protein, phytosterol, amino acid, and metabolite compositions.[45,98] Thus, providing diverse forage for bee pollinators is essential.

Honey bee colonies used for crop pollination often face nutritional stress, because the quality or quantity of pollen forage available to them in such agricultural landscapes can be inadequate.[63] Some cropping systems may put bees at risk for temporary nutritional insufficiency if the crop plant's pollen is deficient in certain nutrients, and bees are unable to find an alternative source of these nutrients. Hence, it is imperative for beekeepers and crop producers to understand the pollen abundance and diversity that honey bees encounter during crop pollination to mitigate nutritional deficiencies by providing supplemental forage[99] (**Fig. 6**). Furthermore, it has been documented that the honey bee colonies used for pollination in certain crops, such as blueberry, exhibit high rates of the bacterial disease European foulbrood (EFB). It is thought that poor foraging, weather, and poor availability of food resources lead to nutritional stress in colonies placed in blueberry fields due to collection of low amounts of food resources (pollen and nectar), which in turn make colonies more susceptible to EFB.

SUMMARY AND FUTURE RESEARCH NEEDS

Honey bee colonies are complex and dynamic biological systems with nutritional needs that change based on internal colony conditions (eg, brood, age of adult bees) and resources that change with exterior/environmental conditions (eg, season, distance, water/drought), with needs and resources not always aligning.[1–5]

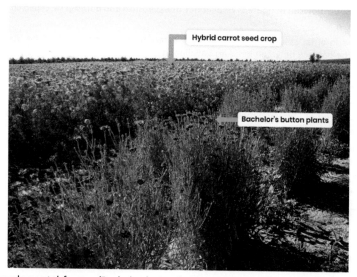

Fig. 6. Supplemental forage (Bachelor button) adjacent to hybrid carrot seed crop.

Pollen and nectar are the primary food resources collected by honey bees. The honey bee colonies depend on these resources not only for colony growth but also to mitigate pathogen infection and expression of detoxification genes.[38,100,101] During resource (pollen and nectar) dearth, beekeepers provide nutritional supplements (protein and sugar) to their colonies. There is a significant gap in knowledge regarding nutritional needs of honey bees, especially micronutrients. Over the past few years, however, there has been renewed focus on understanding the nutrient requirements of honey bees. Many studies related to nutrition are conducted in controlled settings with limited choices for the bees to reduce extraneous variables, whereas in a natural setting, honey bees have several forage options to balance their dietary needs. Hence, there is need for more research in realistic field settings for a robust understanding of honey bee nutritional requirements.

In addition, habitat planting has also become a popular way to improve bee health, but recommendations of floral species are mostly limited to relative attractiveness rather than actual nutritional value. The lack of a current database of floral nutrient values is one challenge that researchers are working to address, but it will take time to build such a database because honey bees are generalists and visit diverse floral species. Continuing research on honey bee nutritional needs and foraging will assist in improving honey bee dietary supplements, habitat recommendations, and colony management.

CLINICS CARE POINTS

- Honey bee nutrition is complex and unique and is not analogous to that of other livestock/animals
- Different life stages of honey bee have different nutritional needs
- Honey bee nutrition is highly dependent on the foraging environment (floral composition of the landscape), and honey bees encounter dynamically changing floral resources in the landscape.
- Optimal nutrition can mitigate several honey bee parasites and pathogens, especially the EFB disease.
- Both the internal colony environment and external environment should be assessed to ensure the balance between need and availability.
- Beekeepers can provide supplemental nutrition (protein and sugars) to their colonies during foraging dearth.
- Caution should be exercised when feeding food resources (honey and pollen) from colonies that have died of unknown reasons or of unknown sources, because some honey bee diseases are transmissible through contaminated food.
- Planting floral habitats is another way to supplement nutrition, but more research is needed to understand the nutritional qualities of different floral resources
- At present, there is a paucity of peer-reviewed published research regarding the benefits of commercial probiotics to honey bees.

DISCLOSURE

The authors have no conflicts of interest and no disclosures to make.

SUPPLEMENTARY DATA

Supplementary data related to this article can be found online at https://doi.org/10.1016/j.cvfa.2021.06.006.

REFERENCES

1. Brodschneider R, Crailsheim K. Nutrition and health in honey bees. Apidologie 2010;41:278–94.
2. Leach ME, Drummond F. A review of native wild bee nutritional health. Int J Ecol 2018;1–10.
3. Donkersley P, Rhodes G, Pickup RW, et al. Honeybee nutrition is linked to landscape composition. Ecol Evol 2014;4:4195–206.
4. Rivera MD, Donaldson-Matasci M, Dornhaus A. Quitting time: When do honey bee foragers decide to stop foraging on natural resources? Front Ecol Evol 2015;3:50.
5. Di Pasquale G, Alaux C, Le Conte Y, et al. Variations in the availability of pollen resources affect honey bee health. PLOS ONE 2016;11:e0162818.
6. Free JB. Factors determining the collection of pollen by honeybee foragers. Anim Behav 1967;15:134–44.
7. Huang ZY, Robinson G. Regulation of honey bee division of labor by colony age demography. Behav Ecol Sociobiol 1996;39:147–58.
8. Tsuruda JM, Page RE. The effects of young brood on the foraging behavior of two strains of honey bees (*Apis mellifera*). Behav Ecol Sociobiol 2009;64:161–7.
9. Sagili RR, Pankiw T, Metz BN. Division of Labor Associated with Brood Rearing in the Honey Bee: How Does It Translate to Colony Fitness? PLOS ONE 2011; 6(2):e16785.
10. Page RE, Fondrk MK. The effects of colony-level selection on the social organization of honey bee (*Apis mellifera* L.) colonies: colony-level components of pollen hoarding. Behav Ecol Sociobiol 1995;36:135–44.
11. Schmickl T, Crailsheim K. Costs of Environmental Fluctuations and Benefits of Dynamic Decentralized Foraging Decisions in Honey Bees. Adapt Behav 2004;12(3–4):263–77.
12. Hellmich RL II, Kulincevic JM, Rothenbuhler WC. Selection for high and low pollenhoarding honey bees. J Hered 1985;76:155–8.
13. Hunt GJ, Amdam GV, Schlipalius D, et al. Behavioral genomics of honeybee foraging and nest defense. Naturwissenschaften 2007;94(4):247–67.
14. Page RE, Amdam GV. The making of a social insect: developmental architectures of social design. BioEssays 2007;29(4):334–43.
15. Tsuruda JM, Amdam GV, Page RE. Sensory response system of social behavior tied to female reproductive traits. PLOS ONE 2008;3:e3397.
16. Wang Y, Kaftanoglu O, Siegel AJ, et al. Surgically increased ovarian mass in the honey bee confirms link between reproductive physiology and worker behavior. J Insect Physiol 2010;56(12):1816–24.
17. Ruedenauer FA, Spaethe J, Leonhardt SD. Hungry for quality—individual bumblebees forage flexibly to collect high-quality pollen. Behav Ecol Sociobiol 2016; 70:1209–17.
18. Pernal SF, Currie RW. The influence of pollen quality on foraging behavior in honeybees (*Apis mellifera* L.). Behav Ecol Sociobiol 2001;51(1):53–68.
19. Beekman M, Preece K, Schaerf TM. Dancing for their supper: Do honeybees adjust their recruitment dance in response to the protein content of pollen? Insect Soc 2016;63:117–26.

20. Corby-Harris V, Snyder L, Meador C, et al. Honey bee (*Apis mellifera*) nurses do not consume pollens based on their nutritional quality. PLOS ONE 2018;13(1): e0191050.

21. Ghosh S, Jeon H, Jung C. Foraging behaviour and preference of pollen sources by honey bee (*Apis mellifera*) relative to protein contents. J Ecol Environ 2020; 44:4.

22. Sagili RR, Pankiw T. Effects of protein-constrained brood food on honey bee (*Apis mellifera* L.) pollen foraging and colony growth. Behav Ecol Sociobiol 2007;61:1471-8.

23. von Frisch K. The dance language and orientation of bees. Cambridge (MA): Harvard University Press; 1967.

24. Couvillon MJ, Riddell Pearce FC, Accleton C, et al. Honey bee foraging distance depends on month and forage type. Apidologie 2015;46:61-70.

25. Danner N, Molitor AM, Schiele S, et al. Season and landscape composition affect pollen foraging distances and habitat use of honey bees. Ecol Appl 2016;26:1920-9.

26. Schmidt-Hempel P. Efficient Nectar-Collecting by Honeybees I. Econ Model. J Anim Ecol 1987;56:209-18.

27. Stabentheiner A, Kovac H. Honeybee economics: optimisation of foraging in a variable world. Sci Rep 2016;6:28339.

28. Heinrich B. Thermoregulation of African and European Honeybees During Foraging, Attack, and Hive Exits and Returns. J Exp Biol 1979;80:217-29.

29. Woods WA, Heinrich B, Stevenson RD. Honeybee flight metabolic rate: does it depend upon air temperature? J Exp Biol 2005;208:1161-73.

30. Schmickl T, Crailsheim K. Inner nest homeostasis in a changing environment with special emphasis on honey bee brood nursing and pollen supply. Apidologie 2004;35:249-63.

31. Couvillon MJ. The dance legacy of Karl von Frisch. Insect Soc 2012;59:297-306.

32. Sponsler DB, Matcham EG, Lin C-H, et al. Spatial and taxonomic patterns of honey bee foraging: A choice test between urban and agricultural landscapes. J Urban Ecol 2017;3:1-7.

33. Nürnburger F, Keller A, Härtel S, et al. Honey bee waggle dance communication increases diversity of pollen diets in intensively managed agricultural landscapes. Mol Ecol 2019;28:3602-11.

34. Wenner AM. Honey bees: do they use the distance information contained in their dance maneuver? Science 1967;155:847-9.

35. Farina WM, Arenas A, Díaz PC, et al. Learning of a mimic odor within beehives improves pollination service efficiency in a commercial crop. Curr Biol 2020;30: 4284-90.e5.

36. Seeley TD. The honey bee colony as a superorganism. Am Sci 1989;77:546-53.

37. Di Pasquale G, Salignon M, Le Conte Y, et al. Influence of Pollen Nutrition on Honey Bee Health: Do Pollen Quality and Diversity Matter? PLOS ONE 2013; 8:e72016.

38. Mao W, Schuler MA, Berenbaum MR. Honey constituents up-regulate detoxification and immunity genes in the western honey bee *Apis mellifera*. Proc Natl Acad Sci USA 2013;110:8842-6.

39. Simone-Finstrom M, Li-Byarlay H, Huang MH, et al. Migratory management and environmental conditions affect lifespan and oxidative stress in honey bees. Sci Rep 2016;6:32023.

40. DeGrandi-Hoffman G, Chen Y, Rivera R, et al. Honey bee colonies provided with natural forage have lower pathogen loads and higher overwinter survival than those fed protein supplements. Apidologie 2016;47:186–96.

41. Glavinic U, Stanovic B, Draskovic V, et al. Dietary amino acid and vitamin complex protects honey bee from immunosuppression caused by *Nosema ceranae*. PLOS ONE 2017;12:e0187726.

42. Mattila HR, Otis GW. Effects of pollen availability and Nosema infection during the spring on division of labor and survival of worker honey bees (Hymenoptera: Apidae). Environ Entomol 2006;35:708–17.

43. Scofield HN, Mattila HR. Honey bee workers that are pollen stressed as larvae become poor foragers and waggle dancers as adults. PLOS ONE 2015;10(4): e0121731.

44. Vaudo AD, Tooker JF, Patch HM, et al. Pollen Protein: Lipid Macronutrient Ratios May Guide Broad Patterns of Bee Species Floral Preferences. Insects 2020; 11(2):132.

45. Chakrabarti P, Morré JT, Lucas HM, et al. The omics approach to bee nutritional landscape. Metabolomics 2019;15:127.

46. Smith CR, Anderson KE, Tillberg CV, et al. Caste determination in a polymorphic social insect: nutritional, social, and genetic factors. Am Nat 2008;172:497–507.

47. Oddo LP, Piazza MG, Pulcini P. Invertase activity in honey. Apidologie 1999; 30(1):57–65.

48. Doner LW. The sugars of honey - a review. J Sci Food Agric 1977;28:443–56.

49. Hrassnigg N, Crailsheim K. Differences in drone and worker physiology in honeybees (*Apis mellifera* L.). Apidologie 2005;36:255–77.

50. Standifer LN. Honey Bee Nutrition and Supplemental Feeding. Beekeeping in the United States, Agriculture Handbook Number 335 1980;39–45.

51. Huang Z. Feeding honey bees. Michigan State University Extension Bulletin E-3369. 2018;1-3.

52. Roulston TH, Cane JH, Buchmann SL. What governs protein content of pollen: pollinator preferences, pollen–pistil interactions, or phylogeny? Ecol Monogr 2000;70:617–43.

53. DeGroot AP. Protein and amino acid requirements of the honeybee (*Apis mellifica* L.). Physiol Comp Oecol 1953;3:197–285.

54. Singh RP, Singh PN. Amino acid and lipid spectra of larvae of honey bee (*Apis cerana* Fabr) feeding on mustard pollen. Apidologie 1996;27:21–8.

55. Schmidt LS, Schmidt JO, Rao H, et al. Feeding preference of young worker honey bees (Hymenoptera: Apidae) fed rape, sesame, and sunflower pollen. J Econ Entomol 1995;88:1591–5.

56. Ellis A, Ellis JD, O'Malley MK, et al. The benefits of pollen to honey Bees. ENY152 Entomology and Nematology Department. Gainesville (FL): UF/IFAS Extension; 2020.

57. Crailsheim K, Schneider LHW, Hrassnigg N, et al. Pollen consumption and utilization in worker honeybees (*Apis mellifera carnica*): dependence on individual age and function. J Insect Physiol 1992;38:409–19.

58. Knecht D, Kaatz HH. Patterns of larval food production by hypopharyngeal glands in adult worker honey bees. Apidologie 1990;21:457–68.

59. Kunert K, Crailsheim K. Seasonal Changes in Carbohydrate, Lipid and Protein Content in Emerging Worker Honeybees and their Mortality. J Apic Res 1988; 27:13–21.

60. Malone LA, Tregidga EL, Todd JH, et al. Effects of ingestion of a biotin-binding protein on adult and larval honey bees. Apidologie 2002;33:447–58.

61. Sagili RR, Metz BN, Lucas HM, et al. Honey bees consider larval nutritional status rather than genetic relatedness when selecting larvae for emergency queen rearing. Sci Rep 2018;8:7679.

62. Keller I, Fluri P, Imdorf A. Pollen nutrition and colony development in honey bees, Part II. Bee World 2005;86:27–34.

63. Naug D. Nutritional stress due to habitat loss may explain recent honeybee colony collapses. Biol Conserv 2009;142:2369–72.

64. DeGrandi-Hoffman G, Chen Y, Huang E, et al. The effect of diet on protein concentration, hypopharyngeal gland development and virus load in worker honey bees (Apis mellifera L.). J Insect Physiol 2010;56:1184–91.

65. Szczesna T. Long chain fatty acids composition of honeybee-collected pollen. J Apic Sci 2006;50(2):65–79.

66. Komosinska-Vassev K, Olczyk P, Kaźmierczak J, et al. Bee pollen: chemical composition and therapeutic application. Evidence-Based Complement Altern Med 2015;2015:297425.

67. Muth F, Breslow PR, Masek P, et al. A pollen fatty acid enhances learning and survival in bumblebees. Behav Ecol 2018;29(6):1371–9.

68. Arien Y, Dag A, Zarchin S, et al. Omega-3 deficiency impairs honey bee learning. Proc Natl Acad Sci USA 2015;112(51):15761–6.

69. Vanderplanck M, Zerck PL, Lognay G, et al. Generalized host-plant feeding can hide sterol-specialized foraging behaviors in bee-plant interactions. Ecol Evol 2020;10(1):150–62.

70. Dobson HEM. Survey of pollen and pollenkitt lipids—chemical cues to flower visitors? Am J Bot 1988;75:170–82.

71. Behmer ST, Nes WD. Insect Sterol Nutrition and Physiology: A Global Overview. Adv Insect Phys 2003;31:1–72.

72. Carvalho M, Schwudke D, Sampaio JL, et al. Survival strategies of a sterol auxotroph. Development 2010;137:3675–85.

73. Herbert EW Jr, Svoboda JA, Thompson MJ, et al. Sterol utilization in honey bees fed a synthetic diet: effects on brood rearing. J Insect Physiol 1980;26:287–9.

74. Feldlaufer MF. Biosynthesis of makisterone A and 20-hydroxyecdysone from labeled sterols by the honey bee. Arch Insect Biochem Physiol 1986;3:415–21.

75. Chakrabarti P, Lucas HM, Sagili RR. Novel Insights into Dietary Phytosterol Utilization and Its Fate in Honey Bees (Apis mellifera L.). Molecules 2020;25:571.

76. Svoboda JA, Thompson MA, Herbert EW, et al. Utilization and Metabolism of Dietary Sterols in the Honey Bee and the Yellow Fever Mosquito. Lipids 1982;17:220–5.

77. Svoboda JA, Herbert EW, Thompson MJ, et al. Selective sterol transfer in the honey bee: Its significance and relationship to other hymenoptera. Lipids 1986;21:97–101.

78. Chakrabarti P, Lucas HM, Sagili RR. Evaluating effects of a critical micronutrient (24-methylenecholesterol) on honey bee physiology. Ann Entomol Soc Am 2019; 113(3):176–82.

79. Chakrabarti P, Sagili RR. Changes in Honey Bee Head Proteome in Response to Dietary 24-Methylenecholesterol. Insects 2020;11:743.

80. Liao L-H, Wu W-Y, Berenbaum MR. Behavioral responses of honey bees (Apis mellifera) to natural and synthetic xenobiotics in food. Sci Rep 2017;7(1):15924.

81. Palmer-Young EC, Tozkar ÖC, Schwarz RS, et al. Nectar and Pollen Phytochemicals Stimulate Honey Bee (Hymenoptera: Apidae) Immunity to Viral Infection. J Econ Entomol 2017;110(5):1959–72.

82. Palmer-Young EC, Farrell IW, Adler LS, et al. Chemistry of floral rewards: intra- and interspecific variability of nectar and pollen secondary metabolites across taxa. Ecol Monogr 2019;89(1):e01335.

83. Johnson RM, Dahlgren L, Siegfried BD, et al. Acaricide, fungicide and drug interactions in honey bees (*Apis mellifera*). PLOS ONE 2013;8(1):e54092.

84. Bernkalu E, Bjostad L, Hogeboom A, et al. Dietary Phytochemicals, Honey Bee Longevity and Pathogen Tolerance. Insects 2019;10(1):14.

85. Saffari A, Kevan PG, Atkinson JL. Consumption of three dry pollen substitutes in commercial apiaries. J Apic Sci 2010;54(2):13–20.

86. Al-Ghamdi AA, Al-Khaibari AM, Omar MO. Consumption rate of some proteinic diets affecting hypopharyngeal glands development in honeybee workers. Saudi J Biol Sci 2011;18(1):73–7.

87. Waller GD, Caron DM, Loper GM. Pollen patties maintain brood rearing when pollen is trapped from honey bee colonies. Am Bee J 1981;122:101–3.

88. Van der Steen J. Effect of a home-made pollen substitute on honey bee colony development. J Apic Res 2007;46:2.

89. Sagili RR, Breece CR. Effects of Brood Pheromone (SuperBoost) on Consumption of Protein Supplement and Growth of Honey Bee (Hymenoptera: Apidae) Colonies During Fall in a Northern Temperate Climate. J Econ Entomol 2012; 105(4):1134–8.

90. Topitzhofer E, Breece C, Wyns D, et al. Honey bee colony maintenance expenses: supplemental feed, requeening and medication. Corvallis (OR): Oregon State University Extension Article PNW 745; 2020. p. 1–7.

91. Romero S, Nastasa A, Chapman A, et al. The honey bee gut microbiota: strategies for study and characterization. Insect Mol Biol 2019;28(4):455–72.

92. Moran NA. Genomics of the honey bee microbiome. Curr Opin Insect Sci 2015; 10:22–8.

93. Lee FJ, Rusch DB, Stewart FJ, et al. Fermentation by honey bee gut microbes. Environ Microbiol 2015;17:796–815.

94. Engel P, Martinson VG, Moran NA. Functional diversity within the simple gut microbiota of the honey bee. Proc Natl Acad Sci USA 2012;109:11002–7.

95. Decourtye A, Mader E, Desneux N. Landscape enhancement of floral resources for honey bees in agro-ecosystems. Apidologie 2010;41:264–77.

96. Lundin O, Ward KL, Artz DR, et al. Wildflower Plantings Do Not Compete With Neighboring Almond Orchards for Pollinator Visits. Environ Entomol 2017; 46(3):559–64.

97. Carroll MJ, Meikle WG, McFrederick QS, et al. Pre-almond supplemental forage improves colony survival and alters queen pheromone signaling in overwintering honey bee colonies. Apidologie 2018;49(6):827–37.

98. Villette C, Berna A, Compagnon V, et al. Plant Sterol Diversity in Pollen from Angiosperms. Lipids 2015;50(8):749–60.

99. Topitzhofer E, Lucas H, Chakrabarti P, et al. Assessment of pollen diversity available to honey bees (Hymenoptera: Apidae) in major cropping systems during pollination in the western United States. J Econ Entomol 2019;112(5):2040–8.

100. Giacomini JJ, Leslie J, Tarpy DR, et al. Medicinal value of sunflower pollen against bee pathogens. Sci Rep 2018;8:14394.

101. Li J, Heerman MC, Evans JD, et al. Pollen reverses decreased lifespan, altered nutritional metabolism and suppressed immunity in honey bees (*Apis mellifera*) treated with antibiotics. J Exp Biol 2019;222:jeb202077.

Honey Bee (*Apis mellifera*) Immunity

Nuria Morfin, PhD[a],*, Ricardo Anguiano-Baez, DVM, MSc[b], Ernesto Guzman-Novoa, PhD[c]

KEYWORDS

- Honey bees • *Apis mellifera* • Defense mechanisms • Innate immunity
- Cellular immunity • Humoral immunity • Social immunity

KEY POINTS

- The innate immunity of honey bees operates through cellular and humoral mechanisms.
- Cellular immunity is governed by hemocytes and includes processes of phagocytosis, nodulation, encapsulation, and melanization.
- Humoral immunity is regulated by Toll, Imd, Jak/Stat, and JNK signaling pathways and culminates with the synthesis of antimicrobial peptides (AMPs).
- RNAi is an important antiviral mechanism.
- Social defense mechanisms include the use of propolis, grooming and hygienic behaviors, and bee fever.

INTRODUCTION

Honey bees (*Apis mellifera*) are arguably the most beneficial of all insects due to their valuable pollinating services for agricultural crops and wild plants, which contribute to human and livestock food production and to the maintenance of ecosystems.[1] However, honey bee colonies have been collapsing at unprecedented rates in recent years, in part due to their increasing exposure to multiple pathogens and other stressors.[2,3]

Honey bees are able to reduce the impact of biotic and abiotic stressors by activating their immune system, responding to these stressors. Many characteristics of the honey bee immune system are shared with other insects, like *Drosophila melanogaster* (fruit fly), *Anopheles gambiae* (malaria mosquito), *Aedes aegypti* (yellow fever mosquito), *Bombyx mori* (silkworm), and *Manduca sexta* (tobacco hornworm), which have been used as models to describe immune responses.[4] Although insects lack

[a] Research Associate, University of Guelph, School of Environmental Sciences, 50 Stone Road East, N1G 2W1, Guelph, Ontario, Canada; [b] Adjunct Professor, National Autonomous University of Mexico, Av. Universidad #3000, CU, Coyoacán, 04510, Mexico City, Mexico; [c] Professor and Head of the Honey Bee Research Centre, University of Guelph, School of Environmental Sciences, 50 Stone Road East, N1G 2W1, Guelph, Ontario, Canada
* Corresponding author.
E-mail address: nmorfinr@uoguelph.ca
Twitter: @MorfinNuria; @HBRC1 (N.M.); @richybat (R.A.-B.)

Vet Clin Food Anim 37 (2021) 521–533
https://doi.org/10.1016/j.cvfa.2021.06.007
0749-0720/21/© 2021 Elsevier Inc. All rights reserved.
vetfood.theclinics.com

adaptive immunity, they have evolved an effective innate immunity, which operates through cellular and humoral responses against pathogens and other stressors[5] (**Fig. 1**). Cellular and humoral immune responses are activated by pathogen recognition molecular patterns (PAMPs), which are highly conserved domains present in pathogens and parasites.[6] PAMPs are recognized by receptors located in the insect's body cells and hemocytes, called pattern recognition receptors (PRRs). Cellular immunity is mediated by hemocytes, which are cells present in the hemolymph, an extracellular fluid that acts as the major transport medium for the nutrients and other molecules in insects.[7] Cellular immune responses include phagocytosis, nodulation, encapsulation, and melanization.[8] Humoral immunity is mediated by the immune deficiency (Imd), Toll, Janus kinase-signal transducer and activator of transcription (Jak/Stat), and c-Jun N-terminal kinase (JNK) pathways,[9] which can result in the synthesis of antimicrobial compounds, like antimicrobial peptides (AMPs), defensive enzymes, and complement-like proteins.[10,11] The antiviral defense mechanisms of honey bees include RNA interference (RNAi), a conserved biological response to double-stranded RNA (dsRNA) that inhibits the expression of protein-coding genes.[12,13]

As social insects, honey bees have evolved other defense mechanisms against diseases and pests, such as the collection of propolis (plant resins with antimicrobial properties) and the removal of diseased brood and parasites by expressing hygienic and grooming behaviors.[14] Honey bees may also increase the temperature of the brood nest (bee fever) to reduce the virulence of microorganisms.[14] Understanding the underlying mechanisms of individual immune responses and social defense behaviors is critical for the development of strategies aimed at reducing the impact of pathogens and other stressors on honey bee health.

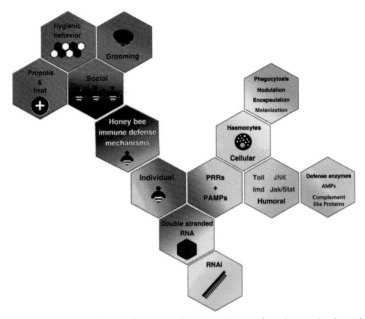

Fig. 1. Summary of honey bee defense mechanisms. Honey bee immunity is activated by PRRs' recognition of PAMPs. Cellular immunity is governed by hemocytes and involves processes of phagocytosis, nodulation, encapsulation, and melanization. Humoral immunity is regulated by signaling pathways (Toll, JNK, Imd, Jak/Stat). Antiviral defense mechanisms include RNAi. Honey bee social immunity includes the use of propolis and the expression of grooming and hygienic behaviors.

ACTIVATION OF IMMUNE RESPONSES

The innate immune system of insects is able to recognize small molecular motifs of pathogens, PAMPs (also known as microbe-associated molecular patterns), such as lipopolysaccharides, lipoteichoic acid, zymosan, flagellin, glycolipids, and glyco-proteins.[6] The innate immune system is also able to identify damage-associated molecular patterns (DAMPs), which are endogenous molecules released from damaged cells.[15] In addition, dsRNA can be identified by the host as a non-sequence-specific virus-associated molecular pattern (VAMPs), triggering antiviral defense mechanisms in the honey bee.[16]

CELLULAR IMMUNITY

Cellular defense mechanisms are mediated by hemocytes and consist of phagocy-tosis, nodulation, encapsulation, clot formation, and melanization (**Fig. 2**).[17–19] Pro-hemocytes in *Drosophila melanogaster* are produced in the procephalic mesoderm during embryogenesis and in the lymphatic gland during the larval stage.[20] Before the lymphatic gland degenerates during pupation, prohemocytes are released into circulation.[20] The prohemocytes produced during the embryogenesis and larval stages contribute to the adult hemocyte population and are differentiated into plas-matocytes, crystal cells, and lamellocytes.[7] Recent studies have identified hemato-poietic hubs in *D melanogaster* adults, located in the dorsal side of the insect's abdomen.[21] During the insect's adult life, hemocytes move with the hemolymph (circulating hemocytes) or are attached to tissues (sessile hemocytes).[8] Hemocytes have been described in different insects based on morphology and function, but the nomenclature of hemocyte populations is not standardized across the order Insecta.[18,22] Negri and colleagues[18] classified honey bee hemocytes based on morphology, in vitro functional descriptions, and locomotion and described 2 types of hemocytes in fifth instar larvae and 4 types of hemocytes in newly emerged worker bees; similarities between honey bee and lepidopteran (butterflies and moths) hemo-cytes were found. The most common types of hemocytes described in the order Insecta are prohemocytes, granulocytes, plasmatocytes, spherulocytes, and eono-cytoids.[17] Gábor and colleagues[23] found that plasmatocytes were the most abun-dant hemocyte subpopulation in honey bees, and unlike *Drosophila*, honey bees had a lower proportion of phagocytic cells.

Hemocyte counts have been used as an indicator of immunocompetence in honey bees. For example, bees parasitized by *Varroa destructor* (varroa mites) had low numbers of hemocytes[24] and bees challenged with *Spiroplasma melliferum* showed a transient hemocyte increase.[25]

Phagocytosis

Phagocytosis is the engulfment of molecules into a nascent organelle of an individual phagocytic cell and occurs after a PRR on the cell surface binds to a PAMP.[8] PRRs involved in phagocytosis are evolutionarily conserved protein families, and the classes include scavenger receptors, fibrinogen-related proteins, Nimrod proteins, Down syn-drome cell adhesion molecules, and peptidoglycan recognition proteins (PGRPs).[22,26,27] However, phagocytic receptors can bind directly to ligands expressed on the surface of target cells or recognize opsonins attached to microor-ganisms or damaged cells.[28] Upon ligand recognition, phagocytic receptors can acti-vate downstream signaling pathways to regulate phagocytosis and also to activate humoral signaling pathways, like Toll.[29]

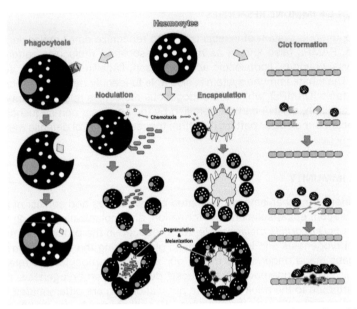

Fig. 2. Summary of honey bee cellular responses. Cellular immunity is mediated by hemocytes and consists of processes of phagocytosis, nodulation, encapsulation, clot formation, and melanization.

Nodulation and Encapsulation

Nodulation and encapsulation are cellular defense mechanisms, characterized by a quick recruitment of hemocytes to contain the damage inflicted by mechanical injuries, to prevent the penetration of pathogens into the insect's body, and to neutralize microorganisms or parasites.[7,8,17] Nodulation occurs in response to the recognition of nonself molecules, such as bacteria, fungi, and protozoa, whereas encapsulation happens as a response to larger invaders, like parasites.[8] These processes start with the penetration of the pathogen into the host and the recognition of PAMPs and DAMPs by PRRs, followed by the chemotaxis of hemocytes to the site of penetration or the location of the pathogen.[30,31] The neutralization of the invader occurs by the degranulation of hemocytes through the activation of serine proteases that cleave prophenoloxidase to generate activated phenoloxidase (PO). PO oxidizes phenols to produce quinones, which polymerize the pigment melanin.[32] Melanin, and the intermediates produced during its formation, such as reactive oxygen species and reactive nitrogen species, are toxic to parasites, bacteria, fungi, and viruses.[29,32]

Hemocytes are also important for coagulation and wound healing.[17] Clot formation consists of the deposition of fibrous matrix, cross-linking proteins, and melanin.[8,17]

HUMORAL IMMUNITY

Humoral responses are regulated by the intracellular signaling pathways Toll, Imd, Jak/Stat, and JNK and culminate with the synthesis of AMPs (**Fig. 3**). AMPs are highly preserved proteins of 12 to 50 amino acids, which are released into the hemolymph after their synthesis in the fat body, integument, and gut epithelial tissues, during bacterial, fungal, or viral infections.[10,11,33]

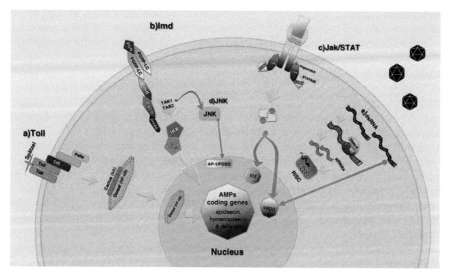

Fig. 3. Immune signaling pathways of honey bees. The activation of (*a*) Toll (*b*) Imd (*c*) Jak/Stat (*d*) JNK (*e*) dsRNA upon recognition of PAMPs, DAMPs, and VAMPs by PRRs culminate in the expression of AMPs-coding genes, like *apidaecin, hymenoptaecin,* and *defensin,* and immune-related genes, like *vago.* (Broderick NA, Welchman, DP, Lemaitre B. Recognition and response to microbial infection in Drosophila. In: Rolff J, Reynolds SE, editors. Insect Infection and Immunity. New York: Oxford University Press.)

Gene expression analysis in honey bees challenged with pathogens or abiotic stressors has been used to assess their humoral immunocompetence. For example, *V. destructor* parasitism and *Nosema ceranae* infection downregulate immune-related genes.[34,35] Also, abiotic stressors, like insecticides and acaricides, affect the regulation of genes coding for AMPs.[34,36] In addition, the combined effect of abiotic and biotic stressors on honey bee humoral responses has been evidenced,[35,37] indicating that honey bees may be immunocompromised by the interaction of stressors.

Toll Pathway

The Toll pathway is activated by the recognition of gram-positive bacteria and fungi.[38] Toll is a transmembrane receptor composed of an ectodomain of leucine-rich repeats (LRRs) and an intracellular Toll/interleukin-1 receptor domain (TIR).[38] Toll is activated by the proteolytic cleavage of Spätzel, a Toll ligand cytokine.[39] Upon activation, Toll recruits TIR and other adaptors to activate the kinase Pelle, which leads to the proteosomal degradation of Cactus (a nuclear factor [NF]-κB inhibitor), facilitating the nuclear translocation of the NF-κB transcriptional factor, Dorsal (the Rel protein Dif is also translocated in *D melanogaster*), inducing the expression of immune genes by binding to κB DNA motifs.[38,40,41]

The Toll signaling pathway has been thoroughly studied in *D melanogaster*, which shows similarities with honey bees. For example, 2 *Spätzel* orthologues and 2 homologues of *dorsal* were found in the honey bee genome.[26] Also, intracellular components that are possibly involved in the Toll pathway have been identified in honey bees, such as Tollip, Pellino, Cactin, and TNF receptor-associated factor-2 (TRAF-2), but further studies are needed to determine their roles in immune responses regulated by the

Toll signaling pathway. The AMPs synthesized by honey bees after the activation of Toll include defensin and drosomycin.[26,36] Evidence of the involvement of Toll in melanization processes has been reported in *D melanogaster* and *Tenebrio molitor* (mealworm), showing a complex interaction between cellular and humoral immunities,[42,43] which should be further investigated in honey bees.

Imd and Jak/Stat Pathways

The Imd pathway is activated after the recognition of gram-negative and gram-positive bacteria with diaminopimelic acid-type peptidoglycans, by PGRP-LC.[44] The Imd cascade occurs by the interaction between the Imd protein and the adaptor dFADD to recruit the caspase Dredd, which is associated with the NF-κB-like transcription factor, Relish.[45] Relish is phosphorylated by the inhibitory κB kinase (IKK) signaling complex, possibly regulated by the kinases TGFβ, TGFβ-associated kinase 1 (TAK1), and TGF-beta-activated kinase 1 (TAB2).[46] Imd also regulates the JNK pathway. For example, the degradation of TAK1 by Relish leads to the termination of the JNK signaling.[47]

Jak/Stat regulates immune responses, homeostatic mechanisms, cell growth, cell differentiation, and apoptosis.[48] Jak/Stat core components in *Drosophila* include 3 ligands called Unpaired (Udp, Udp2, and Udp3), which bind to the Domeless (Dome) receptor and induce the phosphorylation of the cytoplasmic tail of the Dome receptor by JAK tyrosine kinase Hopscotch, to create sites for the latent STAT92E proteins.[48,49] STAT92E proteins are phosphorylated, dimerized, and translocated into the nucleus, where they bind to palindromic response elements to induce gene expression.[48,49] The Jak/Stat pathway in *Drosophila* also regulates the expression of *Turandot* (*Tot*) genes, which are expressed as a result of severe stress,[4] and is involved in antiviral defense mechanisms characterized by an upregulation of immune-related genes, like *vago*.[50] Evans and colleagues[26] found orthologue genes for major components of the Imd and Jak/Stat pathways in honey bees, including *Dome, hopscotch*, and *STAT92E*. However, the ligand *Udp* and *Tot* factors have not been found in the honey bee genome.[26] Honey bees seem to have approximately one-third of the immune-related genes of Toll, Imd, and Jak/Stat pathways compared with other insect genomes,[26] but the implications of these differences remain unknown. Although the Jak/Stat pathway is highly conserved among insects, more studies are needed to characterize the core components of honey bees.

JNK Pathway

The JNK is a conserved mitogen-activated protein kinase (MAPK) pathway, involved in several biological processes, such as embryonic development, apoptosis, stress response, cell proliferation, cell differentiation, and immune responses triggered by gram-negative bacteria.[47,51,52] The JNK pathway branches out from the Imd pathway at dTAK1 and consists of the gene *bsk* and 2 JNK kinases, *Hemipterous* (*hep*) and *DJun/DFos*, which activate the transcription factors AP-1 (Jun/Fos heterodimers) and Forkhead Box O transcription factor FOXO.[51] Immune responses by JNK include the antimicrobial responses regulated by Udp3, Relish, the phosphatase gene *Puckered* (*Puc*), and the Pvr receptor tyrosine kinase.[47,53,54]

ANTIVIRAL DEFENSE MECHANISMS

Different mechanisms are involved in the defense of insects against viral infections, including the Toll, Imd, and JNK signaling pathways, as well as cellular mechanisms like endocytosis.[55–57] However, RNAi and non-sequence-specific dsRNA-mediated antiviral response seem to play a major role in the antiviral mechanisms of honey bees.[13,16]

The antiviral defense mechanisms through the RNAi pathway initiates when the RNAse III family ribonuclease Dicer-2 detects and cleaves viral dsRNA into short viral RNAs (siRNAs). siRNA is loaded into Argonaute-2 (Ago-2), which is the catalytic component of the RNA-induced silencing complex (RISC).[58] One of the siRNA strands, the siRNA guide strand, remains associated with Ago2 and is methylated on its 3' terminal by the methyltransferase Hen1, generating an active RISC.[58] The siRNA guide strand binds to a complementary target single-stranded RNA (ssRNA) leading to the cleavage (silencing) of the target viral ssRNA.[58] The second siRNA strand, the passenger siRNA strand, is degraded in a process that depends on Ago2 and the endoribonuclease C3PO.[59] Moreover, dsRNA is able to trigger nonspecific antiviral defense responses acting as a VAMP and activating signal transduction pathways and the expression of immune-related genes, like *vago*.[16,50]

Studies on RNAi in honey bees have evidenced the role of RNAi on viral defense mechanisms against Israeli acute paralysis virus.[60,61] Also, Desai and colleagues[62] reported that bees fed with dsRNA specific to deformed wing virus (DWV) reduced viral levels in challenged bees. Moreover, Brutscher and colleagues[63] found an upregulation of genes associated with the Toll, Imd, and Jak/Stat pathways in bees infected with Sindbis virus (SINV-GFP), including *hopscotch*, *toll-10*, *tube*, *pirk*, and *jra*, and reported differentially expressed genes coding for AMPs and genes involved in stress responses, like *apidaecin*, *hymenoptaecin*, *abaecin*, *defensin*, *heat shock*, *dicer*, and *vago*. However, Brustcher and collegues[63] found several uncharacterized genes, suggesting that more studies on viral defense mechanisms and gene characterization in honey bees are needed.

SOCIAL IMMUNITY

Honey bees are social insects that have evolved collective defense mechanisms against parasites, which result from the cooperation of individual members of the colony to reduce disease transmission.[14] These collective defense mechanisms may be induced by the presence of pathogens or may be constantly present in the colony and include grooming and hygienic behaviors, bee fever, the use of propolis, and absconding.[14]

Grooming Behavior

Grooming behavior of honey bees involves the use of legs and mandibles for the removal of dustlike materials and ectoparasites from their bodies. There are 2 major categories of bee's grooming behavior: self-grooming (also known as autogrooming) and intergrooming (also known as allogrooming).[64] Self-grooming behavior is effective at removing pollen grains and restraining *V. destructor* and *Acarapis woodi* (tracheal mites) population growth.[65,66] Intergrooming is characterized by the performance of a grooming dance by a bee to get assistance from nestmates to remove particles or parasites, like *V. destructor*, from their bodies.[64]

Honey bee genotypes vary in their ability to express grooming behavior. For example, Africanized honey bees (descendants of *A mellifera scutellata*) are more effective at removing mites from their bodies compared with European bees.[66] The variability in grooming ability among different bee strains is partially affected by genetic effects. The influence of specific genes on honey bee grooming behavior was reported by Arechavaleta-Velasco and collegues[67] who identified a single chromosomal region containing 27 genes associated with self-grooming, including *atlastin*, *ataxin*, and *neurexin-1*. The gene *neurexin* has been associated with intense grooming behavior in response to *V. destructor* parasitism.[68] Traits associated with self-grooming behavior, like mite population growth, number of fallen mites, and the proportion of fallen injured mites, have been used to select honey bees resistant to *V. destructor*.[69,70] Although grooming behavior is regulated by genetic factors,[71] it is also influenced by environmental variables.[72] The ability of the bees to self-groom could also be impacted by the exposure to neurotoxins and parasites.[35] Further information on the molecular regulatory aspects of grooming would benefit breeding programs, which could be incorporated into beekeeping operations to decrease the negative effects of parasites potentially resulting in decreased honey bee mortality.

Hygienic Behavior

Hygienic behavior is the ability of worker adult bees to detect diseased or parasitized brood (larvae or pupae) and uncap the cells to remove their unhealthy contents.[73] Hygienic behavior may control viral, bacterial, and fungal infections, as well as *V. destructor* parasitism.[73–76] Genotypic and phenotypic variability between honey bee strains and maternal effects in the inheritance of hygienic behavior were reported by Unger and Guzman-Novoa.[77] Moreover, 6 or 7 quantitative trait loci (QTL) were found associated with hygienic behavior.[78,79] Tsuruda and colleagues[80] identified 2 QTLs associated with the Varroa sensitive hygiene (VSH) trait, which is a form of hygienic behavior wherein bees identify and remove larvae and pupae infested with reproductive *V. destructor* mites.[81] Spivak and colleagues[82] found that bees expressing hygienic behavior had increased expression of octopamine gene, a neuromodulator that plays a role in olfactory-based behaviors. As with grooming, hygienic behavior could be affected by neurotoxins, such as insecticides and acaricides,[83,84] potentially compromising the ability of the bees to defend themselves against infectious agents and parasites. Selective breeding of bees for hygienic behavior has shown promising results to control brood diseases and parasitism, including American foulbrood and varroosis.[75,85]

Propolis and Other Social Defense Mechanisms

Honey bees collect resins of trees and shrubs (propolis) and use them as prophylactic agents owing to their antimicrobial properties.[14] After collecting propolis, bees coat the interior walls of their nests (propolis envelope) as well as small animals that cannot be carried out of the nest by the bees.[86,87] Hives with a propolis envelope were found to have lower viral levels and lower expression of immune genes, indicating that propolis prevents the dissemination of diseases and contributes to a decrease in the energetic cost of having an active immune system.[87] Moreover, honey bees generate additional heat in the nest to control pathogens, such as the fungus *Ascosphaera apis*,[88] through a mechanism known as bee fever. In addition, honey bees may abscond when the levels of pathogens, parasites, or pests are high, leaving behind brood and food stores. Although absconding could be a mechanism to control diseases in honey bee populations, it is not a desirable trait for profitable beekeeping.[14]

SUMMARY

Honey bees are exposed to biotic and abiotic stressors, which can compromise their health and survival. Honey bees rely on innate immune defense mechanisms to fight diseases through cellular and humoral responses. Comparative studies between honey bees and other insects have shown conserved mechanisms in their innate immune systems, but more studies to identify and characterize components of their immunity are still needed. Hemocyte counts and the expression of immune-related genes have been used to assess immunocompetence in bees, helping elucidate the effect and interaction of stressors on them. A better understanding of the mechanisms underlying immune responses and the interconnections between humoral and cellular pathways would help to implement prophylactic and therapeutic strategies to prevent honey bee mortality and increase their productivity. Moreover, the incorporation of traits associated with social immunity, such as grooming and hygienic behavior, in selective breeding programs has shown promising results for increasing the resistance of bees to diseases and parasites. Further investigations on the molecular mechanisms regulating such traits would greatly benefit breeding programs.

CLINICS CARE POINTS

- The periodic monitoring of the brood chamber allows for the identification of pests and diseases and their timely treatment.
- Following regulatory procedures for the application of agricultural chemicals is essential to prevent the exposure of bees to abiotic stressors that could compromise their immune system.
- The control of *V. destructor* within a colony prevents high viral levels, particularly viruses vectored by *V. destructor* (eg, DWV).
- The incorporation of honey bee stock selected for hygienic and/or grooming behavior is key in an integrated pest management strategy to prevent extreme honey bee colony losses.

DISCLOSURE

The authors have nothing to disclose.

REFERENCES

1. Potts SG, Imperatriz-Fonseca V, Ngo HT, et al. Safeguarding pollinators and their values to human well-being. Nature 2016;540:220–9.
2. vanEngelsdorp D, Meixner MD. A historical review of managed honey bee populations in Europe and the United States and the factors that may affect them. J Invertebr Pathl 2010;103:S80–95.
3. Guzman-Novoa E. Colony collapse disorder and other threats to honey bees. In: Cork S, Hall DC, Liljebjelke K, editors. One health case studies: addressing complex problems in a changing world. Sheffield: 5M Publishing Ltd; 2016. p. 204–16.
4. Broderick NA, Welchman DP, Lemaitre B. Recognition and response to microbial infection in *Drosophila*. In: Rolff J, Reynolds SE, editors. Insect infection and immunity. New York: Oxford University Press; 2009. p. 13–33.
5. Buchmann K. Evolution of innate immunity: clues from invertebrates via fish to mammals. Front Immunol 2014;5:1–8.
6. Wang Q, Ren M, Liu X, et al. Peptidoglycan recognition proteins in insect immunity. Mol Immunol 2019;106:69–76.
7. Klowden MJ. Circulatory systems. In: Physiological systems in insects. Cambridge: Academic press; 2013. p. 365–413.
8. Strand MR. The insect cellular immune response. Insect Sci 2008;15:1–14.
9. Medzhitov R, Janeway CA. Innate immunity: impact on the adaptive immune response. Curr Opin Immunol 1997;9:4–9.

10. Meister M, Lemaitre B, Hoffmann JA. Antimicrobial peptide defense in *Drosophila*. BioEssays 1997;19:1019–26.

11. Huang J-H, Jing X, Douglas AE. The multi-tasking gut epithelium of insects. Insect Biochem Mol Biol 2015;67:15–20.

12. Niu J, Meeus I, Cappelle K, et al. The immune response of the small interfering RNA pathway in the defense against bee viruses. Curr Opin Insect Sci 2014; 6:22–7.

13. Brutscher LM, Daughenbaugh KF, Flenniken ML. Antiviral defense mechanisms in honey bees. Curr Opin Insect Sci 2015;10:71–82.

14. Simone-Finstrom M. Social immunity and the superorganism: behavioral defenses protecting honey bee colonies from pathogens and parasites. Bee World 2017;94:21–9.

15. Nace G, Evankovich J, Eid R, et al. Dendritic cells and damage-associated molecular patterns: endogenous danger signals linking innate and adaptive immunity. JIN 2012;4:6–15.

16. Flenniken ML, Andino R. Non-specific dsRNA-mediated antiviral response in the honey bee. PLoS One 2016;8(10):e77263.

17. Lavine MD, Strand MR. Insect hemocytes and their role in immunity. Insect Biochem Mol Biol 2002;32:1295–309.

18. Negri P, Maggi M, Szawarski N, et al. *Apis mellifera* haemocytes *in-vitro*, What type of cells are they? Functional analysis before and after pupal metamorphosis. J Apic Res 2014;53:576–89.

19. Marringa WJ, Krueger MJ, Burritt NL, et al. Honey bee hemocyte profiling by flow cytometry. PLoS One 2014;9:e108486.

20. Lanot R, Zachary D, Holder F, et al. Postembryonic hematopoiesis in *Drosophila*. Dev Biol 2001;230:243–57.

21. Ghosh S, Singh A, Mandal S, et al. Active hematopoietic hubs in drosophila adults generate hemocytes and contribute to immune response. Dev Cell 2015; 33:478–88.

22. Hillyer JF. Insect immunology and hematopoiesis. Dev Comp Immunol 2016;58: 102–18.

23. Gábor E, Cinege G, Csordás G, et al. Identification of reference markers for characterizing honey bee (*Apis mellifera*) hemocyte classes. Dev Comp Immunol 2020;19:103701.

24. Koleoglu G, Goodwin PH, Reyes-Quintana M, et al. *Varroa destructor* parasitism reduces hemocyte concentrations and prophenol oxidase gene expression in bees from two populations. Parasitol Res 2018;117:1175–83.

25. Yang D, Zha G, Li X, et al. Immune responses in the haemolymph and antimicrobial peptide expression in the abdomen of *Apis mellifera* challenged with *Spiroplasma melliferum* CH-1. Microb Pathog 2017;112:279–87.

26. Evans JD, Aronstein K, Chen YP, et al. Immune pathways and defence mechanisms in honey bees *Apis mellifera*. Insect Mol Biol 2006;15:645–56.

27. Nazario-Toole AE, Wu LP. Chapter two - phagocytosis in insect immunity. In: Ligoxygakis P, editor. Advances in insect physiology (Insect immunity), vol 52. Cambridge: Academic Press; 2017. p. 35–82.

28. Ratcliffe NA, Rowley AF. Opsonic activity of insect hemolymph. In: Cheng TC, editor. Invertebrate blood: cells and serum factors (Comparative pathobiology). New York: Springer US; 1984. p. 187–204.

29. Nakhleh J, El Moussawi L, Osta MA. Chapter three - the melanization response in insect immunity. In: Ligoxygakis P, editor. Advances in insect physiology (Insect immunity), vol 52. Cambridge: Academic Press; 2017. p. 83–109.

30. Wood W, Faria C, Jacinto A. Distinct mechanisms regulate hemocyte chemotaxis during development and wound healing in *Drosophila melanogaster*. J Cell Biol 2006;173:405–16.
31. Ling E, Shirai K, Kanekatsu R, et al. Hemocyte differentiation in the hematopoietic organs of the silkworm, *Bombyx mori*: prohemocytes have the function of phagocytosis. Cell Tissue Res 2005;320:535–43.
32. Binggeli O, Neyen C, Poidevin M, et al. Prophenoloxidase activation is required for survival to microbial infections in drosophila. PLoS Pathog 2014;10:e1004067.
33. Huang X, Xu Y, Zhang Y, et al. Spatzle4 gene of silkworm, *Bombyx mori*: Identification, immune response, and the effect of RNA interference on the antimicrobial peptides' expression in the integument. Saudi J Biol Sci 2018;25:1817–25.
34. Garrido PM, Porrini MP, Antúnez K, et al. Sublethal effects of acaricides and *Nosema ceranae* infection on immune related gene expression in honeybees. Vet Res 2016;47:51.
35. Morfin N, Goodwin PH, Hunt GJ, et al. Effects of sublethal doses of clothianidin and/or *V. destructor* on honey bee (*Apis mellifera*) self-grooming behavior and associated gene expression. Sci Rep 2019;9:5196.
36. Di Prisco G, Cavaliere V, Annoscia D, et al. Neonicotinoid clothianidin adversely affects insect immunity and promotes replication of a viral pathogen in honey bees. PNAS 2013;110:18466–71.
37. Tesovnik T, Cizelj I, Zorc M, et al. Immune related gene expression in worker honey bee (*Apis mellifera carnica*) pupae exposed to neonicotinoid thiamethoxam and Varroa mites (*Varroa destructor*). PLoS One 2017;12:e0187079.
38. Valanne S, Wang J-H, Rämet M. The *Drosophila* Toll signaling pathway. J Immunol 2011;186:649–56.
39. Arnot CJ, Gay NJ, Gangloff M. Molecular mechanism that induces activation of spätzle, the ligand for the drosophila toll receptor. J Biol Chem 2010;285:19502–9.
40. Belvin MP, Jin Y, Anderson KV. Cactus protein degradation mediates *Drosophila* dorsal-ventral signaling. Genes Dev 1995;9:783–93.
41. Hetru C, Hoffmann JA. NF-κb in the immune response of *Drosophila*. Cold Spring Harb Perspect Biol 2009;1:a000232.
42. Kan H, Kim C-H, Kwon H-M, et al. Molecular control of phenoloxidase-induced melanin synthesis in an insect. J Biol Chem 2008;283:25316–23.
43. Dudzic JP, Hanson MA, Iatsenko I, et al. More than black or white: melanization and Toll share regulatory serine proteases in *Drosophila*. Cell Rep 2019;27:1050–61.e3.
44. Yu Y, Park J-W, Kwon H-M, et al. Diversity of innate immune recognition mechanism for bacterial polymeric meso-diaminopimelic acid-type peptidoglycan in insects. J Biol Chem 2010;285:32937–45.
45. Stöven S, Ando I, Kadalayil L, et al. Activation of the *Drosophila* NF-κB factor Relish by rapid endoproteolytic cleavage. EMBO Rep 2000;1:347–52.
46. Ertürk-Hasdemir D, Broemer M, Leulier F, et al. Two roles for the *Drosophila* IKK complex in the activation of Relish and the induction of antimicrobial peptide genes. PNAS 2009;106:9779–84.
47. Park JM, Brady H, Ruocco MG, et al. Targeting of TAK1 by the NF-κB protein Relish regulates the JNK-mediated immune response in *Drosophila*. Genes Dev 2004;18:584–94.
48. Bang IS. JAK/STAT signaling in insect innate immunity. Entomol Res 2019;49:339–53.

49. Bina S, Zeidler M. JAK/STAT pathway signalling in *Drosophila melanogaster*. In: Stephanou A, editor. JAK-STAT pathway in disease (Madame curie bioscience database). Texas: Landes Bioscience; 2009. p. 2000–13.

50. Deddouche S, Matt N, Budd A, et al. The DExD/H-box helicase Dicer-2 mediates the induction of antiviral activity in *Drosophila*. Nat Immunol 2008;9:1425–32.

51. Delaney JR, Stöven S, Uvell H, et al. Cooperative control of *Drosophila* immune responses by the JNK and NF-κB signaling pathways. EMBO J 2006;25:3068–77.

52. Tafesh-Edwards G, Eleftherianos I. JNK signaling in *Drosophila* immunity and homeostasis. Immunol Lett 2020;226:7–11.

53. McEwen DG, Peifer M. Puckered, a *Drosophila* MAPK phosphatase, ensures cell viability by antagonizing JNK-induced apoptosis. Development 2005;132: 3935–46.

54. Bond D, Foley E. A quantitative RNAi screen for JNK modifiers identifies *pvr* as a novel regulator of *Drosophila* immune signaling. PLoS Pathog 2009;5:e1000655.

55. Costa A, Jan E, Sarnow P, et al. The IMD pathway is involved in antiviral immune responses in *Drosophila*. PLoS One 2009;4:e7436.

56. Nakamoto M, Moy RH, Xu J, et al. Virus recognition by toll-7 activates antiviral autophagy in *Drosophila*. Immunity 2012;36:658–67.

57. Chowdhury A, Modahl CM, Tan ST, et al. JNK pathway-a key mediator of antiviral immunity in mosquito salivary glands. Access Microbiol 2019;1:88.

58. Hammond SM, Boettcher S, Caudy AA, et al. Argonaute2, a link between genetic and biochemical analyses of RNAi. Science 2001;93:1146–50.

59. Liu Y, Ye X, Jiang F, et al. C3PO, an endoribonuclease that promotes RNAi by facilitating RISC activation. Science 2009;325:750–3.

60. Maori E, Paldi N, Shafir S, et al. IAPV, a bee-affecting virus associated with Colony Collapse Disorder can be silenced by dsRNA ingestion. Insect Mol Biol 2009;18: 55–60.

61. Hunter W, Ellis J, vanEngelsdorp D, et al. Large-scale field application of RNAi technology reducing Israeli acute paralysis virus disease in honey bees (*Apis mellifera*, hymenoptera: apidae). PLoS Pathog 2010;6:e1001160.

62. Desai SD, Eu Y-J, Whyard S, et al. Reduction in deformed wing virus infection in larval and adult honey bees (*Apis mellifera* L.) by double-stranded RNA ingestion. Insect Mol Biol 2012;21:446–55.

63. Brutscher LM, Daughenbaugh KF, Flenniken ML. Virus and dsRNA-triggered transcriptional responses reveal key components of honey bee antiviral defense. Sci Rep 2017;7:6448.

64. Pritchard DJ. Grooming by honey bees as a component of varroa resistant behavior. J Apic Res 2016;55:38–48.

65. Danka RG, Villa JD. Autogrooming by resistant honey bees challenged with individual tracheal mites. Apidologie 2003;34:591–6.

66. Guzman-Novoa E, Emsen B, Unger P, et al. Genotypic variability and relationships between mite infestation levels, mite damage, grooming intensity, and removal of *Varroa destructor* mites in selected strains of worker honey bees (*Apis mellifera* L.). J Invertebr Pathol 2012;110:314–20.

67. Arechavaleta-Velasco ME, Alcala-Escamilla K, Robles-Rios C, et al. Fine-scale linkage mapping reveals a small set of candidate genes influencing honey bee grooming behavior in response to varroa mites. PLoS One 2012;e47269.

68. Hamiduzzaman MM, Emsen B, Hunt GJ, et al. Differential gene expression associated with honey bee grooming behavior in response to varroa mites. Behav Genet 2017;47:335–44.

69. Hunt GJ, Given K, Tsuruda MJ, et al. Breeding mite-biting bees to control *Varroa*. Bee Cult 2016;8:41–7.
70. Morfin N, Given K, Evans M, et al. Grooming behavior and gene expression of the Indiana "mite-biter" honey bee stock. Apidologie 2020;51:267–75.
71. Moretto G, Gonçalves L, De Jong D. Heritability of Africanized and European honey bee defensive behavior against the mite *Varroa jacobsoni*. Rev Bras Genet 1993;16:71–7.
72. Currie RW, Tahmasbi GH. The ability of high- and low-grooming lines of honey bees to remove the parasitic mite *Varroa destructor* is affected by environmental conditions. Can J Zool 2008;1059–67.
73. Rothenbuhler WC. Behavior genetics of nest cleaning in honey bees. IV. responses of F1 and backcross generations to disease-killed blood. Am Zool 1964;4:111–23.
74. Gilliam M, Taber S, Richardson GV. Hygienic behavior of honey bees in relation to chalkbrood disease. Apidologie 1983;14:29–39.
75. Spivak M, Reuter GS. Resistance to American foulbrood disease by honey bee colonies *Apis mellifera* bred for hygienic behavior. Apidologie 2001;32(6):555–65.
76. Vung NN, Choi YS, Kim I. High resistance to Sacbrood virus disease in *Apis cerana* (Hymenoptera: Apidae) colonies selected for superior brood viability and hygienic behavior. Apidologie 2020;51:61–74.
77. Unger P, Guzman-Novoa E. Maternal effects on the hygienic behavior of Russian × Ontario hybrid honeybees (*Apis mellifera* L). J Hered 2010;101:91–6.
78. Lapidge KL, Oldroyd BP, Spivak M. Seven suggestive quantitative trait loci influence hygienic behavior of honey bees. Naturwissenschaften 2002;89:565–8.
79. Oxley PR, Spivak M, Oldroyd BP. Six quantitative trait loci influence task thresholds for hygienic behaviour in honeybees (*Apis mellifera*). Mol Ecol 2010;19:1452–61.
80. Tsuruda JM, Harris JW, Bourgeois L, et al. High-resolution linkage analyses to identify genes that influence varroa sensitive hygiene behavior in honey bees. PLoS One 2012;7:e48276.
81. Harris JW, Danka RG, Villa JD. Honey bees (hymenoptera: apidae) with the trait of Varroa sensitive hygiene remove brood with all reproductive stages of varroa mites (Mesostigmata: Varroidae). Ann Entomol Soc Am 2010;103:146–52.
82. Spivak M, Masterman R, Ross R, et al. Hygienic behavior in the honey bee (*Apis mellifera* L.) and the modulatory role of octopamine. J Neurol 2003;55:341–54.
83. Morfin N, Goodwin PH, Correa-Benitez A, et al. Sublethal exposure to clothianidin during the larval stage causes long-term impairment of hygienic and foraging behaviours of honey bees. Apidologie 2019;50:595–605.
84. Gashout HA, Guzman-Novoa E, Goodwin PH. Synthetic and natural acaricides impair hygienic and foraging behaviors of honey bees. Apidologie 2020. https://doi.org/10.1007/s13592-020-00793-y.
85. Danka RG, Harris JW, Dodds GE. Selection of VSH-derived "Pol-line" honey bees and evaluation of their Varroa-resistance characteristics. Apidologie 2016;47:483–90.
86. Ghisalberti EL. Propolis: A review. Bee World 1979;60:59–84.
87. Borba RS, Wilson MB, Spivak M. Hidden benefits of honeybee propolis in hives. In: Vreeland RH, Sammataro D, editors. Beekeeping – from science to practice. Berlin: Springer International Publishing; 2017. p. 17–38.
88. Starks PT, Blackie CA, Seeley TD. Fever in honeybee colonies. Naturwissenschaften 2000;87:229–31.

Practical Applications of Genomics in Managing Honey bee Health

Tanushree Tiwari, PhD Candidate, Amro Zayed, PhD*

KEYWORDS

- Haplodiploidy • Polyandry • SNP • Genome-wide association studies
- Transcriptome • Biomarkers

KEY POINTS

- Genome-wide association studies are opening the door to improving bee health via marker-assisted selection.
- Single-nucleotide polymorphism genotyping is critical for stopping the transmission of invasive bee species.
- Discovering stressor-specific biomarkers from expression profiling can be used to diagnose why colony health declines in the field.

INTRODUCTION

The honey bee *Apis mellifera* is a model organism for the study of social behavior and is essential to our agroeconomy because of its importance to pollination. The honey bee is the most widely used pollinator in agriculture because their large perennial colonies can be moved wherever they are needed, enabling beekeepers and farmers to easily deploy large numbers of bees for pollination whenever necessary. However, honey bee colonies have experienced declining health leading to colony losses over the past 2 decades. For example, the average winter mortality in Canada and the United States over the past decade is 24.3%[1] and 27.3%,[2] respectively. These averages are higher than the historic threshold of 15% mortality experienced by North American beekeepers before the introduction of *Varroa* mites. Some specific years have been extremely challenging for North American beekeepers. In 2020, the Canadian winter mortality averaged 30.2%,[1] with some provinces reporting even higher values. Similarly, beekeepers in the United States lost approximately 43.7% of their colonies in the winter of 2020. This loss is the second highest average annual loss

a Department of Biology, York University, 208 Lumbers Building, 4700 Keele Street, Toronto, Ontario M3J 1P3, Canada
* Corresponding author.
E-mail address: zayed@yorku.ca

Vet Clin Food Anim 37 (2021) 535–543
https://doi.org/10.1016/j.cvfa.2021.06.008
0749-0720/21/© 2021 Elsevier Inc. All rights reserved.

in the United States, with the first occurring earlier this decade in 2013 when approximately 45% of colonies died during the winter.[3] These losses are unsustainable and have the potential to negatively impact our agroeconomy and our food security.

Broadly speaking, several general factors have been implicated in the decline of honey bee health. These factors are commonly called the 4 "P's": Pathogens, Pests, Pesticides, and Poor nutrition.[4] Stressors, however, do not act in isolation, and their interactions are difficult to predict. For example, pesticides used in agriculture can act synergistically rather than having additive effects on honey bees.[5] Pesticide exposure and nutritional stress in the form of limited forage on monoculture can compromise the honey bee's immune response, making them more susceptible to parasites.[4] It is clear that chronic exposure to multiple interacting stressors is an important factor leading to honey bee colony losses and declines of wild pollinators, but the combination and number of stressors differ from place to place,[6] making universal diagnoses and cures for bee health very challenging.

Managed honey bee populations are also at risk from hybridization with invasive honey bee lineages, such as "killer" bees in South America and clonal bees in South Africa. "Killer bees," hybrid African and west European bees accidently introduced to South America in 1956,[7] are up to 6 times more defensive (ie, aggressive) than European-derived bees.[8] Their swarming frequency is also high, which, combined with their aggression, make them very difficult to manage commercially. Similarly, parasitic clonal bees from the cape of South Africa, *Apis mellifera capensis*, can wreak havoc on commercial managed honey bees, leading to dwindling colony syndrome.[9] These workers invade colonies and produce clonal female offspring through automixis,[10] thereby establishing themselves as pseudo queens; once established, these clonal workers continue reproducing until the colony collapses.[11]

The study of honey bee genetics and genomics offers many intriguing possibilities for improving honey bee health. The first honey bee genome was sequenced in 2006.[12] This genome sequence was assembled with DNA extracted from multiple drones derived from a single queen.[12] A more contiguous genome assembly of *A mellifera* was released in 2019[13] using a combination of data from long-read and short-read sequencing. The long reads played a significant role in filling the gaps and joining thousands of scaffolds into 16 superscaffolds. The newer assembly particularly improved the quality of the bee genome near repetitive regions.[13] Overall, the honey bee genome contains ∼236 million base-pairs organized into 16 chromosomes with more than 10,000 predicted genes.[12] The size of the bee genome is one-tenth that of the human genome.

Several properties render honey bees different for most typical livestock from a genetics and breeding perspective. Honey bees are haplodiploid[14]: females are diploid, and males are haploid. The sex of a bee is determined by genotype at a variable autosomal gene known as complementary sex determiner, *csd*.[14] Queen bees can selectively fertilize their eggs. Unfertilized eggs are hemizygous at *csd*, and these eggs develop into haploid males.[15] When producing daughters or future queens, females will fertilize their eggs and under most circumstances (because of the high genetic variability at *csd*), and these eggs will be heterozygous at *csd* and develop as female.[14] However, under some circumstances, fertilized eggs will be homozygous at *csd*, leading to the development of diploid males, which are eaten by workers at the first larval instar stage.[16] Any population genetic process that leads to a reduction in genetic diversity at *csd*, such as low effective population size or inbreeding, will result in higher frequencies of diploid male production, leading to a phenotype called "shot brood", a very spotty brood pattern, as many of the developing larva are removed by workers[14]; this phenomena drains the colony of workers and substantially reduces the colony's fitness.[17] As such, many of the classical selective breeding methods applied to livestock cannot be effectively applied to honey bees.

In addition to haplodiploidy, queen honey bees are highly polyandrous.[18] Queens naturally mate with a large number of haploid males (typically, 15–25 males) during the first week of their life as adults and store the sperm for use over the duration of their lifespan (2–4 years), introducing a high degree of genetic diversity within colonies, which has been linked to colony fitness.[19] Polyandry also makes traditional breeding approaches common in other livestock very difficult because of our general inability to control mating. Although it is possible to use instrumental insemination to generate desired crosses,[20] the technique requires highly specialized skill sets and equipment and is not commonly used in beekeeping.

Last, a major difficulty with studying honey bee genetics is that many of the traits of interest are "collective" and are thus not directly amenable to genetic experiments aimed at studying traits expressed by individuals. A honey bee colony contains a single reproductive queen and thousands of sterile workers (ie, nurses, foragers, guards) that build and maintain the nest, care for the brood, forage for food, and engage in nest defense.[21] Worker bees exhibit many fascinating behaviors, such as dancing to communicate the location of new food sources,[22] removing sick or dead individuals from a hive to prevent the spread of disease,[23] attacking invaders,[24] grooming each other to remove pests and parasites,[25] and clustering together in the winter to keep the colony warm.[26] These collective behaviors, performed by a large number of cooperating workers with different genetics, ultimately contribute to the survival of colonies. Elucidating the genetics of these colony level traits has been challenging.

Despite the difficulties introduced by haplodiploidy, *csd*, polyandry, and sociality, there is substantive potential for using genetics and genomics in managing bee health. Here, the authors review 3 practical applications of incorporating genomics into everyday beekeeping. First, they discuss the utility of using single-nucleotide polymorphisms (SNPs) to distinguish between the many European and Asian honey bee subspecies that are commonly used in apiculture and invasive strains that are undesirable for beekeeping. Second, many honey bee traits are highly heritable and can thus be improved by selective breeding. The authors discuss the potential for using genomics to identify causal mutations underlying economically valuable traits and using them in marker-assisted selection (MAS). Finally, when honey bee colonies perish, it is often very difficult to understand the specific causes that led to their demise. The authors discuss the potential of using expression biomarkers to rapidly identify stressors affecting honey bee colonies in the field.

APPLICATION 1: STOCK CERTIFICATION AND CONTROL OF INVASIVE LINEAGES

The availability of honey bee genomes and SNP data sets has allowed us to identify genomic variation within and between populations or species of honey bees.[27–29] These studies help in elucidating differences in genetics between native honey bee subspecies and the source and contribution of these native subspecies in the typically highly admixed managed colonies used in beekeeping.[30–33] Diagnostic mutations for specific honey bee races can be used in breeding programs aimed at maintaining pure local subspecies, which are at risk of extinction via introgression with managed honey bees.[34,35] Moreover, several studies have identified sets of SNPs that are successful in separating managed honey bees from invasive Africanized "killer" bees. For example, a diagnostic assay of 95[36] and 37[37] SNPs has been developed to accurately identify "killer bees" by measuring their African lineage ancestry. These diagnostic assays should be widely used to ascertain the genetics of imported queens or colonies, especially in North America, where killer bees are spreading into areas with large queen breeding operations in the southern United States.[38,39]

APPLICATION 2: MARKER ASSISTED SELECTION POWERED BY GENOME-WIDE ASSOCIATION STUDIES

Many of the colony level traits that influence the health and temperament of honey bee colonies are heritable. For example, narrow-sense heritability for hygienic behavior, a type of social immunity whereby hygienic bees uncap and remove dead or *Varroa*-infected pupae from the colony, is between 20% and 65%.[40,41] Similarly, honey production by a colony is an economically important trait that beekeepers wish to maximize and has a heritability ranging from 25% to 60%.[42] Defensive behavior is a colony-level heritable trait whereby guard bees detect intruders at the colony entrance and release alarm pheromones, which recruits older bees that sting intruders, sacrificing themselves in the process.[43] Heritability estimates for defensive behavior range between 13% and 43%.[44] The temperament of bees is important for the industry, as beekeepers generally prefer to work with docile bees.[45,46] In addition, at the individual level, honey bees have several lines of innate immune defense mechanisms against pathogens, and it is known that some of these defenses are heritable as well. For example, the antimicrobial peptide abaecin has a heritability estimate between 30% and 40%.[47] In theory, this heritability can be used to breed honey bees with superior characteristics for beekeeping.

Population genomics methods are useful in identifying genes and mutations with signatures of natural or artificial selection. Generally, population genomic studies sequence bees that show phenotypic differences caused either by natural selection in native bee races or by artificial selection acting to enhance specific traits in managed populations. Traditional analysis of positive selection[48,49] thereby enables researchers to identify genes and mutations associated with phenotypic traits. For example, a recent study sequenced drones from populations selected for high royal jelly production and discovered 44 regions associated with this trait.[50] Sequencing haploid drones in bees is beneficial because it reduces the sequencing coverage needed to accurately identify SNPs. A similar study sequenced populations selected for high hygienic behavior and identified 73 protein-coding genes associated with this trait.[51]

Genome-wide association studies (GWAS) is an emerging approach for uncovering candidate regions of a genome associated with complex quantitative traits, such as behavior. Powered by next-generation sequencing data, GWAS approaches have made it economically practical and feasible to sequence thousands of individuals to discover millions of common SNPs[52] and associate these genetic differences with phenotypic differences between individuals.[53] Genome-wide association mapping is suitable for identifying common mutations that have small to medium additive effects on a phenotype.[54] A major advantage of GWAS for identifying the loci that affect bee health is that it does not require crosses that are difficult to perform in the honey bee.

Another benefit of applying GWAS in honey bees is that honey bees have very high recombination rates resulting in rapid decay of linkage disequilibrium.[55] This typically results in small genomic regions showing a statistical association with traits studied via GWAS (tens of kilobases or smaller); however, adequately powered experiments are needed to achieve such results.[56] If the causal variants affecting key honey bee traits can be identified, such as immunity, aggression, hygiene, honey production, and overwintering mortality, breeding efforts can be substantially aided by applying MAS.[57]

Although still uncommon, a few GWAS-type studies have been carried out on honey bees. For example, using a 44,000 Affymetrix SNP array, researchers studied a social immune trait involving the detection and uncapping of a *Varroa*-affected brood by honey bee workers and discovered 6 SNP markers for the trait.[58] Recently, a GWAS study was performed to determine the genetics of defensive behavior in honey bees.[59] The investigators found 1172 SNPs for which colony allele frequency was significantly associated with colony defensive behavior.[59] The authors look forward to more GWAS studies on honey bee traits of ecological and economical importance.

APPLICATION 3: BIOMARKERS FOR DIAGNOSING BEE HEALTH

Beekeepers and conservation practitioners do not have adequate diagnostic tools to understand why honey bee health is declining, and this is hampering abilities to manage honey bees and circumvent colony losses. Beekeepers rarely have access to professional support to help them diagnose bee health issues, unlike in other livestock systems. Presently, beekeepers manually inspect colonies and treat them with miticides and antibiotics to manage a few known pests and pathogens, often without knowing or testing their levels. For pathogens, quantitative polymerase chain reaction assays are available,[60] but the testing methods are costly and low throughput. Similarly, analysis of agrochemicals found within bees and colonies is possible but typically is too expensive for regular use in bee health management. Often, beekeepers would only carry out postmortem tests for agrochemicals or pathogens if they experienced unusually high colony mortality, but obviously, postmortem tests are not effective for planning interventions. These shortcomings are creating problems for beekeepers, veterinarians, and government agencies who require real-time data on stressors within colonies to better understand how to manage and improve bee health.

There is a strong need for robust methods to identify stressors impacting the health of bee colonies. Here, biomarker-based assays can play a pivotal role in understanding the stressors affecting colonies. Biomarkers are commonly used in human health care and livestock management[61] for diagnosing disease. A few studies have suggested that expression profiling can be used to identify stressor-specific biomarkers in bees, who have distinct genetic pathways for dealing with pathogenic,[62] nutritional,[63] and xenobiotic[64] challenges that are associated with specific and measurable changes in gene expression. For example, a large meta-analysis of transcriptomic studies involving honey bees exposed to different pests and pathogens discovered both common and pathogen-specific changes in gene expression associated with infections.[65] For example, *Atg2* (LOC726497), *Metap2* (LOC551771), and *Dnr1* (LOC412897) are among genes that were differentially expressed when colonies were exposed to microsporidian parasite, *Nosema* (but not *Varroa* mites), whereas *Iap2* (LOC413374), *Rel* (LOC552247), *Tube* (LOC725368), and *Defensin2* were differentially expressed when colonies had *Varroa* and viral infections (but not *Nosema*). These genes are potential biomarkers for infection by *Nosema* or *Varroa*, respectively.

In theory, a comprehensive set of experiments that expose bees to a large number of relevant stressors, followed by expression profiling, can identify stressor-specific biomarkers that can be used for honey bee health diagnostics. Work on this front has started with the BeeCSI project (https://beecsi.ca/). This project involves assaying the transcriptome, proteome, and gut microbiome of many bees exposed to a variety of pathogenic, xenobiotic, and nutritional stressors in the laboratory and in the field. By comparing lists of differentially expressed markers across studies, the BeeCSI team will strive to identify stressor-specific biomarkers (eg, genes that are upregulated in bees exposed to the insecticide clothianidin) as well as general biomarkers (eg, genes that are upregulated in bees exposed to a general class of insecticides, such as neon-icotinoids). These tools can be used by beekeepers and veterinarians to understand and manage stressors affecting honey bee colonies, or by governmental regulators investigating general patterns affecting bee health at regional, provincial, or national scales.

SUMMARY

Several practical applications have been discussed that can help mitigate honey bee losses and improve bee health. The methods target different aspects of the bee health problem and thus collectively provide a powerful toolkit for improving the genetic stock of managed honey bees and for diagnosing or monitoring the health of colonies in the field. Although these applications have yet to reach maturity in honey bee diagnostics, similar methods and tools have been successfully applied in many livestock systems. With the reduced cost of next-generation sequencing, it is becoming increasingly feasible to perform the discussed analyses on a large number of colonies typically managed by beekeepers for crop pollination, honey production, and queen breeding. The wide adoption and use of these tools will result in improvement of health of managed honey bee colonies like never before.

CLINICS CARE POINTS

- Distinguishing between commonly managed strains of honey bees and more aggressive, invasive lineages can be determined using single-nucleotide polymorphisms.
- Selective breeding and marker-assisted selection are developing fields and have remarkable potential to improve disease management and honey bee health.
- Once expression biomarkers were commercially available, and veterinarians and beekeepers may find expression biomarkers useful in the diagnostic process by rapidly identifying stressors affecting honey bee colonies in the field.
- Although the genomic solutions discussed are still in the developmental stage, veterinarians should keep themselves updated with developments in the ever-changing landscape of bee health and genomics.

DISCLOSURE

We acknowledge funding from Canada's Natural Sciences and Engineering Research Council of Canada and York University's Research Chair program to Amro Zayed.

REFERENCES

1. Ferland J, Kempers M, Kennedy K, et al. Canadian Association of Professional Apiculturists statement on honey bee wintering losses in Canada. 2020;22. Available at: https://capabees.com/shared/CAPA-Statement-on-Colony-Losses-2020.pdf.
2. Bruckner SS, Rennich K, Aurell SD, et al, for the Bee Informed, preliminary PUShbcl. p-rAM. United States honey bee colony losses 2017-2018: preliminary results. 2019. Available at: https://beeinformed.org/results/honey-bee-colony-losses-2017-2018- r, 2019.
3. Bruckner S, Steinhauer N, Rennich K, et al. Honey bee colony losses 2017–2018: preliminary results. Bee Informed Partnership; 2018. Available at: https://

beeinformed.org/2018/06/21/preliminary-results-2017-2018-total-and-average-honey-bee-colony-losses-by-state-and-the-district-of-columbia/.

4. Goulson D, Nicholls E, Botías C, et al. Bee declines driven by combined stress from parasites, pesticides, and lack of flowers. Science 2015;347(6229):1255957.
5. Sih A, Bell AM, Kerby JL. Two stressors are far deadlier than one. Trends Ecology Evolution 2004;19(6):274–6.
6. Neumann P, Carreck NL. Honey bee colony losses. J Apic Res 2010;49(1):1–6.
7. Jernelöv A. African "Killer Bees" in the Americas. In: Jernelöv A, editor. The long-term fate of invasive species. Cham, Switzerland: Springer; 2017. p. 251–60.
8. Stort A, Gonçalves L. The 'African'Honey bee 1991.
9. Allsopp M, Crewe R. The Cape honey bee as a Trojan horse rather than the hordes of Genghis Khan. Am Bee J 1993;133:121–3.
10. Verma S, Ruttner F. Cytological analysis of the thelytokous parthenogenesis in the Cape honey bee (Apis mellifera capensis Escholtz). Apidologie 1983;14(1):41–57.
11. Hemmling C, Koeniger N, Ruttner F. Quantitative Bestimmung der 9-oxodecen-säure im Lebenszyklus der Kapbiene (Apis mellifera capensis Escholtz). Apidologie 1979;10(3):227–40.
12. Consortium HGS. Insights into social insects from the genome of the honey bee Apis mellifera. Nature 2006;443(7114):931.
13. Wallberg A, Bunikis I, Pettersson OV, et al. A hybrid de novo genome assembly of the honey bee, Apis mellifera, with chromosome-length scaffolds. BMC Genomics 2019;20(1):275.
14. Beye M, Hasselmann M, Fondrk MK, et al. The gene csd is the primary signal for sexual development in the honey bee and encodes an SR-type protein. Cell 2003;114(4):419–29.
15. Beye M. The dice of fate: the csd gene and how its allelic composition regulates sexual development in the honey bee, Apis mellifera. Bioessays 2004;26(10):1131–9.
16. Woyke J. What happens to diploid drone larvae in a honey bee colony. J Apic Res 1963;2(2):73–5.
17. Zayed A. Effective population size in Hymenoptera with complementary sex determination. Heredity 2004;93(6):627–30.
18. Tarpy DR, Page J, Robert E. No behavioral control over mating frequency in queen honey bees (Apis mellifera L.): implications for the evolution of extreme polyandry. Am Nat 2000;155(6):820–7.
19. Mattila HR, Seeley TD. Genetic diversity in honey bee colonies enhances productivity and fitness. Science 2007;317(5836):362–4.
20. Cobey SW, Tarpy DR, Woyke J. Standard methods for instrumental insemination of Apis mellifera queens. J Apic Res 2013;52(4):1–18.
21. Michener CD. The social behavior of the bees: a comparative study. Cambridge (MA): Harvard University Press; 1974.
22. Von Frisch K. The dance language and orientation of bees. Cambridge (MA): Belknap Press; 1967.
23. Park O, Pellet F, Paddock F. Disease resistance and American foulbrood. Am Bee J 1937;77(1):20–5.
24. Breed MD, Diaz PH, Lucero KD. Olfactory information processing in honey bee, Apis mellifera, nestmate recognition. Anim Behav 2004;68(4):921–8.
25. Aumeier P. Bioassay for grooming effectiveness towards Varroa destructor mites in Africanized and Carniolan honey bees. Apidologie 2001;32(1):81–90.

26. Seeley TD, Visscher PK. Survival of honey bees in cold climates: the critical timing of colony growth and reproduction. Ecol Entomol 1985;10(1):81–8.
27. Parejo M, Wragg D, Gauthier L, et al. Using whole-genome sequence information to foster conservation efforts for the European Dark Honey Bee, Apis mellifera mellifera. Front Ecol Evol 2016;4:140.
28. Harpur BA, Kent CF, Molodtsova D, et al. Population genomics of the honey bee reveals strong signatures of positive selection on worker traits. Proc Natl Acad Sci U S A 2014;111(7):2614–9.
29. Cornman RS, Boncristiani H, Dainat B, et al. Population-genomic variation within RNA viruses of the Western honey bee, Apis mellifera, inferred from deep sequencing. BMC Genomics 2013;14(1):154.
30. Harpur BA, Minaei S, Kent CF, et al. Management increases genetic diversity of honey bees via admixture. Mol Ecol 2012;21(18):4414–21.
31. Chapman NC, Harpur BA, Lim J, et al. Hybrid origins of Australian honey bees (Apis mellifera). Apidologie 2016;47(1):26–34.
32. Harpur B, Chapman N, Krimus L, et al. Assessing patterns of admixture and ancestry in Canadian honey bees. Insectes Sociaux 2015;62(4):479–89.
33. Harpur BA, Minaei S, Kent CF, et al. Admixture increases diversity in managed honey bees: reply to De la Rúa et al. (2013). Mol Ecol 2013;22(12):3211–5.
34. Henriques D, Parejo M, Vignal A, et al. Developing reduced SNP assays from whole-genome sequence data to estimate introgression in an organism with complex genetic patterns, the Iberian honey bee (Apis mellifera iberiensis). Evol Appl 2018;11(8):1270–82.
35. Muñoz I, Henriques D, Jara L, et al. SNP s selected by information content outperform randomly selected microsatellite loci for delineating genetic identification and introgression in the endangered dark European honey bee (Apis mellifera mellifera). Mol Ecol Resour 2017;17(4):783–95.
36. Chapman NC, Harpur BA, Lim J, et al. A SNP test to identify Africanized honey bees via proportion of 'African' ancestry. Mol Ecol Resour 2015;15(6):1346–55.
37. Chapman NC, Bourgeois AL, Beaman LD, et al. An abbreviated SNP panel for ancestry assignment of honey bees (Apis mellifera). Apidologie 2017;48(6):776–83.
38. Kono Y, Kohn JR. Range and frequency of Africanized honey bees in California (USA). PLoS One 2015;10(9):e0137407.
39. Lin W, McBroome J, Rehman M, et al. Africanized bees extend their distribution in California. PLoS One 2018;13(1):e0190604.
40. Harbo JR, Harris JW. Responses to Varroa by honey bees with different levels of Varroa Sensitive Hygiene. J Apic Res 2009;48(3):156–61.
41. Rothenbuhler WC. Behaviour genetics of nest cleaning in honey bees. I. Responses of four inbred lines to disease-killed brood. Anim Behav 1964;12(4):578–83.
42. Soller M, Bar-Cohen R. Some observations on the heritability and genetic correlation between honey production and brood area in the honey bee. J Apic Res 1967;6(1):37–43.
43. Hunt G. Flight and fight: a comparative view of the neurophysiology and genetics of honey bee defensive behavior. J Insect Physiol 2007;53(5):399–410.
44. Bienefeld K, Pirchner F. Heritabilities for several colony traits in the honey bee (Apis mellifera carnica). Apidologie 1990;21(3):175–83.
45. Hunt GJ, Amdam GV, Schlipalius D, et al. Behavioral genomics of honey bee foraging and nest defense. Naturwissenschaften 2007;94(4):247–67.
46. Breed MD, Robinson GE, Page RE. Division of labor during honey bee colony defense. Behav Ecol Sociobiol 1990;27(6):395–401.

47. Decanini LI, Collins AM, Evans JD. Variation and heritability in immune gene expression by diseased honey bees. J Hered 2007;98(3):195–201.
48. Fuller ZL, Niño EL, Patch HM, et al. Genome-wide analysis of signatures of selection in populations of African honey bees (Apis mellifera) using new web-based tools. BMC Genomics 2015;16(1):1–18.
49. Nielsen R. Molecular signatures of natural selection. Annu Rev Genet 2005;39: 197–218.
50. Wragg D, Marti-Marimon M, Basso B, et al. Whole-genome resequencing of honey bee drones to detect genomic selection in a population managed for royal jelly. Sci Rep 2016;6(1):1–13.
51. Harpur BA, Guarna MM, Huxter E, et al. Integrative genomics reveals the genetics and evolution of the honey bee's social immune system. Genome Biol Evol 2019;11(3):937–48.
52. Koboldt DC, Steinberg KM, Larson DE, et al. The next-generation sequencing revolution and its impact on genomics. Cell 2013;155(1):27–38.
53. Hayes B. Overview of statistical methods for genome-wide association studies (GWAS). In: Gondro, Cedric, van der Werf, et al, editors. Genome-wide association studies and genomic prediction. Totowa (NJ): Humana Press; 2013. p. 149–69.
54. Korte A, Farlow A. The advantages and limitations of trait analysis with GWAS: a review. Plant Methods 2013;9(1):29.
55. Wallberg A, Glémin S, Webster MT. Extreme recombination frequencies shape genome variation and evolution in the honey bee, Apis mellifera. PLoS Genet 2015;11(4):e1005189.
56. Wu Y, Zheng Z, Visscher PM, et al. Quantifying the mapping precision of genome-wide association studies using whole-genome sequencing data. Genome Biol 2017;18(1):1–10.
57. Guarna MM, Hoover SE, Huxter E, et al. Peptide biomarkers used for the selective breeding of a complex polygenic trait in honey bees. Sci Rep 2017;7(1):1–10.
58. Spötter A, Gupta P, Mayer M, et al. Genome-wide association study of a Varroa-specific defense behavior in honey bees (Apis mellifera). J Hered 2016;107(3): 220–7.
59. Avalos A, Fang M, Pan H, et al. Genomic regions influencing aggressive behavior in honey bees are defined by colony allele frequencies. Proc Natl Acad Sci U S A 2020;117(29):17135–41.
60. Evans JD, Schwarz RS, Chen YP, et al. Standard methods for molecular research in Apis mellifera. J Apic Res 2013;52(4):1–54.
61. Adnane M, Kelly P, Chapwanya A, et al. Improved detection of biomarkers in cervicovaginal mucus (CVM) from postpartum cattle. BMC Vet Res 2018;14(1):1–6.
62. Brutscher LM, Daughenbaugh KF, Flenniken ML. Antiviral defense mechanisms in honey bees. Curr Opin Insect Sci 2015;10:71–82.
63. Kunieda T, Fujiyuki T, Kucharski R, et al. Carbohydrate metabolism genes and pathways in insects: insights from the honey bee genome. Insect Mol Biol 2006;15(5):563–76.
64. Claudianos C, Ranson H, Johnson R, et al. A deficit of detoxification enzymes: pesticide sensitivity and environmental response in the honey bee. Insect Mol Biol 2006;15(5):615–36.
65. Doublet V, Poeschl Y, Gogol-Döring A, et al. Unity in defence: honey bee workers exhibit conserved molecular responses to diverse pathogens. BMC Genomics 2017;18(1):207.

Foreign Pests as Potential Threats to North American Apiculture

Tropilaelaps mercedesae, Euvarroa spp, Vespa mandarinia, and Vespa velutina

Samuel D. Ramsey, PhD[a,b,c,d],*

KEYWORDS

- Tropi mites • *Euvarroa sinhai* • *Euvarroa* mites • *Vespa mandarinia*
- Asian giant hornet • Vespa velutina • Yellow-legged hornet, Honey bee disease

KEY POINTS

- The greatest population density of *Apis mellifera* exists in Asia along with many other honey bee species, allowing frequent opportunity for these species to exchange parasites and pathogens.
- *Tropilaelaps mercedesae* is likely to be more destructive to global apiculture than *Varroa destructor*.
- *Euvarroa* are hardy, fecund parasites well able to exploit *A mellifera* but to this point a verified host shift has yet to occur.
- Successful attacks by *Vespa mandarinia* on *A mellifera* invariably result in the destruction of the entire colony unlike attacks by parasites, which a host may survive.
- *V velutina* spread rapidly in ecosystems and have proved difficult to manage via common methods of *Vespa* management.

INTRODUCTION

Fascination with honey bees goes back millennia.[1,2] Owing primarily to their numerous contributions to culture, science, medicine, food production, and industry, honey bees are well known and widely revered. But this attention has focused most consistently on the Western honey bee, *Apis mellifera* Linnaeus, to the extent that most are surprised to find that there are apparently 10 other genetically distinct honey bee

[a] Agricultural Research Service, Bee Research Laboratory, United States Department of Agriculture, 10300 Baltimore Avenue, Building 306, Beltsville, MD 20705, USA; [b] Ramsey Research Foundation, Temple Hills, MD 20748, USA; [c] University of Maryland; [d] Cornell University
* Corresponding author: Bee Research Laboratory, United States Department of Agriculture, 10300 Baltimore Avenue, Building 306, Beltsville, MD 20705.
E-mail address: samuel.ramsey@usda.gov
Twitter: @drsammytweets (S.D.R.)

Vet Clin Food Anim 37 (2021) 545–558
https://doi.org/10.1016/j.cvfa.2021.06.010
0749-0720/21/© 2021 Elsevier Inc. All rights reserved.

species.[3,4] These other species are native to Asia, making it the homeland of honey bee biodiversity.[5] Each species has its own suite of adapted parasites, pathogens, and/or predators.[5,6] As the singular species not from Asia, *A mellifera* developed in the presence of few specialist natural enemies.[6] Having been introduced into Asia, more managed colonies of *A mellifera* exist there than anywhere else in the world, providing constant opportunity for natural enemies of closely related species to make the jump to this biologically naïve host.[6,7] As such, the greatest diversity of biological threats to *A mellifera* exists in Asia, and any attempts to understand emerging biological threats to the Western honey bee likely should start in the east.

Several parasites, pathogens, and specialist predators have made the discovery that, unlike Asian honey bee species, *A mellifera* is lacking in adequate defenses against them.[8–13] As this list grows, it is imperative that understanding of these potential pest organisms grows with it. These natural enemies typically begin to expand their geographic range after making a host shift to *A mellifera*.[14–17] Because *A mellifera* has a nearly cosmopolitan distribution, it can be difficult to manage this spread. As such, efforts to understand these pests must include evaluation of management and eradication methods in the event that a foreign pest should circumvent our best efforts at preventing introduction. Of particular concern is *Tropilaelaps mercedesae* Anderson and Morgan (Tropi mite), *Euvarroa* spp (*Euvarroa* mite), and the hornet species *V mandarinia* Smith (Asian giant hornet [AGH]) and *V velutina* Lepeletier (yellow-legged hornet [YLH]). Each of these species has multiple characteristics of heavily damaging invasive species, and some have already begun to establish invasive populations beyond Asia.[15,17,18]

TROPI MITE: TROPILAELAPS MERCEDESAE
Background

T mercedesae (Tropi or the Tropi mite) is 1 of 4 species of mites in the genus *Tropilaelaps* (the others being *T clareae*, *T koenigerum*, and *T thaii*).[19] Each of these mites is an obligate parasite of honey bees and can be found in association with honey bee colonies across all 3 honey bee subgenera (dwarf bees, giant bees, and cavity-nesting bees). Of the 4 species, 2 (*T mercedesae* and *T clareae*) have shown the ability to successfully parasitize *A mellifera*.[20] These species are closely related and difficult to distinguish from each other, having only recently been resolved as 2 species from the 1 originally proposed.[20] *T mercedesae* was resolved from *T clareae* in 2007 and determined to be the most geographically widespread and economically/ecologically concerning of the species given its expanding geographic/host range. As a result of confusion related to these cryptic species, widespread records of the destructive nature of *T clareae* actually are referring to that of *T mercedesae*.[14] Many publications, records, and regulations still have not been updated with the most recent taxonomical designation.

Like the commonly encountered *Varroa* mite, Tropi are small external parasites measuring close to 1 mm in length and approximately half a millimeter in width.[20] They typically are a reddish-brown color but tend to fade to a dim tan in collections of preserved specimens. Their body shape in combination with long legs distributed in a narrow arc about the body allow for the parasite's characteristic maneuverability and speed.[21] The Tropi mite, having expanded its range beyond Southeast Asia, can be found throughout much of continental Asia from South Korea to Iran.[14,22] Populations also are found commonly in the Oceania nation of Papua New Guinea.[15]

Similar to other *Apis* brood parasites, Tropi mites have 2 unique stages of their lifecycle, designated the reproductive phase and phoretic phase. During their reproductive phase, they invade host brood cells of late-stage larvae and subsequently are sealed inside by attendant nurse bees.[23] Reproduction occurs, to the best of current knowledge, only inside of sealed brood cells. Tropi diverge from the typical brood parasite lifecycle with which most apiculturists are familiar (ie, *Varroa*) in that they often briefly invade cells of fairly young larvae to feed from them as well.[24] This is likely an adaptation to ensure mites have food resources more consistently available to them because they are phoretic in the succeeding stage and, as such, do not derive nutrition from their adult hosts. Their time outside of brood cells is truncated by comparison to other *Apis* brood parasites in that Tropi typically spend only a day in this stage in comparison to the weeks to months shown in *Varroa* and *Euvarroa*.[25,26] This rapid transition back to the reproductive stage allows Tropi to rapidly expand their population levels within a colony (**Figs. 1**A & B).

Impact on Apis mellifera

Tropi mites have proved highly injurious within and outside of their native geographic range.[19,27,28] In Pakistan in the 1980s, beekeepers began to report damage from a mite that they had not seen to that point; later identified as Tropi mites.[29] Having imported *A mellifera* colonies from Australia less than 10 years earlier in an effort to replace *A cerana* beekeeping in the region, the colonies soon were totally wiped out.[27,29] Beekeepers in the region were unfamiliar with modern mite treatments because none were needed when working with *A cerana*.[29] As a result, Tropi mites were able to wipe out the entirety of their beekeeping operation. There likely were other contributing factors in addition to Tropi but still it underscores the impact that these mites can have when their populations are given access unchecked to honey bees in a region. Further destructive impacts to apiculture have been recorded in other regions of its expanded range, including Afghanistan, Papua New Guinea, and China.[15,28,30] Infested colonies suffer precipitative health decline, reduced honey yield, and eventual collapse.[19]

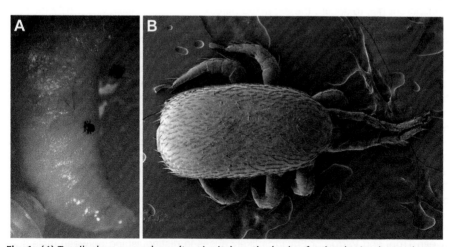

Fig. 1. (*A*) Tropilaelaps mercedesae (tropi mite) on the body of a developing honey bee extracted from a brood cell in an Apis mellifera colony in Northern Thailand. (*B*) Low-Temperature Scanning Electron Micrograph of a tropi mite collected from an apiary in Bangladesh. Note the long front legs used as sensory organs rather than locomotory appendages. The six ambulatory legs are distributed in a narrow arc around the body allowing for rapid locomotion.

Their impact is related broadly to a host of deleterious impacts connected to their feeding behaviors. Tropi chelicera have 2 opposing digits, which the mites use to tear into their host.[31] The ragged holes torn in the host's integument are likely an easy entry point for microorganisms, which then challenge the immune system of the developing bee. Furthermore, Tropi are known to feed on multiple regions of the host's body, inflicting new feeding wounds in subsequent bouts of feeding.[19] This stands in contrast to V destructor, which feeds consistently from 1 wound kept open by the constant revisiting of the population of mites within the cell.[32] It is possible, if not likely, that Tropi feed similarly to V destructor, damaging and consuming fat body tissue, leading to myriad negative health effects.[33] Their feeding results in reduced weight of the eventual adult, reduced protein concentration, and shortened life span.[19] Tropi also are associated with multiple virus that they apparently vector to host bees.[19,34]

Detection/identification

As a result of the Tropi mite's tenuous association with adult bees, there currently is no diagnostic measure able to consistently diagnose the presence of the mites within a colony or the level of brood infestation from a sample of adults. This applies to methods commonly used to detect Varroa, such as alcohol washes and sugar shakes. The brief amount of time spent on the adult population contributes to frequent occurrences where Tropi mites have high levels in brood but very little if any presence on adult bees.[19,35] Add to this their small size, which leaves them just on the margins of human vision, and there is a pest that easily can escape detection. To consistently determine the presence of this species, evaluation of the brood is necessary either by painstaking uncapping of a standard number of brood cells or by means of striking a brood frame against a surface to extract debris from cells. This protocol, referred to as the bump method, may heavily damage brood in the process. It can be conducted more efficiently by scraping away wax broadly from the capping of cells first and then striking the frame against a pan coated in a thin layer of petroleum jelly (or other transparent gel) to secure the extracted mites.

Live specimens of Tropi easily can be distinguished from other similarly sized mites periodically found in honey bee colonies by their movement patterns. Tropi move via sprints interspersed with brief moments of rest similar to the rapid movements of insects like tiger beetles (Coleoptera: Carabidae).[36] Like the tiger beetles, the brief periods of rest may be a necessity of navigating at such speeds with the limits on real-time processing on this small organism's nervous system. The rapid darting movements of Tropi on hive frames easily can distinguish this insect from the slow, lumbering movements of Varroa and Euvarroa mites.

If unable to view the movements, Tropi can be distinguished from other bee mites readily by the trained eye as well, although the aid of a magnifying lens or dissecting scope may be needed. Varroa mites are blood red in coloration and are wider than they are long. Tropi mites by comparison are more pale reddish-brown to tan in coloration and are always longer than they are wide. They usually measure approximately a third the width of Varroa.[14,20] The differences typically are clear if both mites can be compared during the identification process. The most difficulty in distinguishing between Tropi and Varroa or Euvarroa likely arises in distinguishing between male and juvenile forms of Varroa/Euvarroa and Tropi. Male and immature Varroa routinely are mistaken for Tropi under the rare occasions that these reclusive forms are seen outside of a brood cell. Both the adult male and immature stages of Varroa (and ostensibly the closely related Euvarroa) show some superficial similarities to Tropilaelaps in size and shape. Tropi can be distinguished from these mites via attention to coloration.

Adult male *Varroa* and immature mites are pale white and only gain faint color briefly after eating when their diet passes visibly through the digestive system as their integument is transparent.

Management

Much of the impact of this mite on apiculture has been attributed to a lack of effective chemotherapeutics.[15,28] To this point, no chemical measures are registered for usage against this pest. Current efforts to control Tropi mites focus on adapting treatment measures effective against *V destructor* to Tropi. Differences in behavior and lifecycle between the 2 species have stymied some of these efforts. Usage of the common varroacide amitraz (Apistan) has proved ineffective at controlling this species likely because its mode of action is dependent on contact between the mites and active adult bees for extended periods which Tropi mites are uniquely suited to avoid.[37] The chemical flumethrin (in its Bayvarol formulation) has been tested against Tropi mites and in a recent study was proved ineffective at reducing populations likely for similar reasons to the failure seen in amitraz.[15] Systemics distributed within the adult bee population likely would be ineffective at controlling this species because there is no evidence at this point that Tropi mites feed on adult bees.

Wood dowels or commercially available paint stirrers can be soaked in 85% formic acid overnight and applied beneath the frames of a colony as a fumigant. This method has been used by beekeepers in Northern Thailand for several years. Although effective at killing Tropi, this method led to substantial die-off of worker bees when tested in Northern Thailand (Ramsey and colleagues, unpublished data, 2020). A more consistent and controlled means of applying formic acid is Formic Pro or Mite Away Quick Strips. Such a method was tested in the same study and proved similarly effective but without the detrimental impact on the adult bee population. With further refinement, the paint stirrer method potentially could be utilized more effectively by lowering the dosage of formic acid. Usage of heat as a means of controlling Tropi populations showed promise in a preliminary study in Northern Thailand because it resulted in significant reductions in Tropi levels (Ramsey and colleagues, unpublished data, 2020). Furthermore, the removal of brood and destruction of brood from infested colonies is practiced in Thailand as a means of managing Tropi as the mites are dependent on brood for feeding and reproduction.[19]

Clinics Care Points

- Monitoring before and after treatment is essential to confirm that the mite population has not developed resistance to the treatment measure in use.
- Tropi respond best to treatments that have an impact on mites reproducing within capped cells.
- If all else fails, ridding the colony of brood (capped and uncapped) is an effective means of remediation, bringing the colony back to undetectable mite levels quickly.

EUVARROA MITES: *EUVARROA SINHAI* AND *EUVARROA WONGSIRII*
Background

Euvarroa is a genus of parasitic mites composed of 2 species (*E sinhai* Delfinado and Baker and *E wongsirii* Lekprayoon and Tangkanasing) in the family Varroidae.[38] All species within this family are obligate parasites of honey bees, the most infamous of which is *V destructor*. *V destructor* is considered the greatest single contributor to honey bee health decline globally, having achieved a nearly cosmopolitan distribution.[39,40] Similarities in behavior and morphology between *Euvarroa* spp and *V destructor* suggest that *Euvarroa* may be similarly equipped to extensively disrupt global apiculture. *Euvarroa* are found consistently where dwarf honey bees (*A florea* Fabricius and *A andreniformis* Smith) are found. This includes the Malay peninsula, Indonesia, Palawan Island, Indochina, India, and the Middle East.[41]

The *Euvarroa* lifecycle can be divided into 2 stages (reproductive and dispersal) based on the reproductive state of the adult female mite. In the reproductive stage, a female mite known as the foundress invades the brood cell of a late-stage honey bee larva. Soon after, the cell is capped sealing the mite inside with the larva. As the larva begins its transition into its pupal stage, the foundress starts to feed on the immature bee.[26] The female mite lays a single egg at a regular interval and eventually establishes a population of male and female mites within the cell. These mites are able to mate inside of the cell, ensuring that female mites emerge fully capable of becoming foundresses themselves.[17]

Upon emergence, adult female mites move onto the adult bee population (apparently both drones and workers).[17] This period of the lifecycle shows the hardy, long-lived nature of this species by comparison to related species like *T mercedesae*, which can survive on adult bees for less than 2 days before they apparently die of starvation.[42] In *Euvarroa,* the dispersal stage can, reportedly, last for 10 months.[26] The mites use this stage both to disperse to new colonies and to survive periods where the seasonally available drone brood is not present.

Impact on Apis mellifera

The potential impact of *Euvarroa* on *A mellifera* populations is difficult to estimate because little research has been conducted regarding these parasites to date. Furthermore, the fact that no known population has yet transitioned to *A mellifera* makes speculation of impact on the population level that much more challenging. Although the dwarf honey bees (*A florea* and *A andreniformis*) appear minimally impacted by this parasite, the same was the case with Tropi and *Varroa* on their original hosts.[16,19] Now both species are considered extremely deleterious to the Western honey bee.[14,39] Similarities in the morphology of the mouthparts and behavior of *Euvarroa* and *Varroa* suggest common themes in how these species impact their host. In a laboratory setting, Koeniger and colleagues[43] found these parasites beneath the abdominal sternites of adult *A mellifera*. This region was determined to be an important feeding site for access to fat body tissue, the targeted host resource exploited by *V destructor*.[33,44] Thus, it is likely that feeding by the species is similarly injurious to the host.

Euvarroa populations on their original host are restricted to drone brood, which limits their impact on the colony. Such restrictions may change, however, with a host shift. Furthermore, in a laboratory study of *E sinhai* reproducing on worker brood of *A mellifera*, foundress mites produced more than 3 times as many viable offspring in one round of their reproductive stage than *V destructor*.[45] Such similarities to *V destructor* in addition to evidence of a heightened reproductive rate suggest that *Euvarroa* could become a significant stress factor of the Western honey bee.

Detection/identification

Euvarroa are miniscule parasites and, as such, can be difficult to detect in large samples of honey bees. Methods of dislodging similar honey bee ectoparasites like *Varroa* likely would be effective against these mites as well. There methods consist of collecting a standardized sample (typically 100–300 bees) and applying an agent that can disrupt the attachment of the mites to the host bees.[46,47] Powdered sugar, alcohol, and water with detergent added have proved effective in detaching *Varroa*. Powdered sugar can be employed easily in the field for rapid detection and has the added benefit of allowing for the continued survival of the bees in the sample. Alcohol and detergent washes are destructive sampling methods but may yield greater efficiency in circumstances of lower parasite loads. In addition to parasitizing adult bees, *Euvarroa* is a brood parasite and thus can be detected by uncapping sealed brood and conducting a visual inspection of the contents of the cell. Such a method typically is time-consuming but provides accurate resolution of the reproductive population.

Once collected, the parasite must then be accurately identified to species. *Euvarroa* are superficially similar to *Varroa*, which can make this part of the process difficult. *Euvarroa*, however, possess identifying anatomic features best distinguished with the help of a dissecting scope. Among the most conspicuous of these are the long marginal setae extending posteriorly from the posterior margin of the adult female mites. These hairs number between 47 and 54 for *E wongsirii* and 39 and 40 in *E sinhai*.[48,49] They stand in contrast to the short, much thicker irregular setae arising from the lateral margins of the body of *V destructor*. Furthermore, the general body shape for *E sinhai* is rounded and in *E wongsirii* the body has a broad triangular shape in contrast to the ellipsoid shape of *V destructor*.[49,50]

Management

Euvarroa have yet to become pests of the commercially managed honey bee species (*A cerana*, *A indica* Fabricius, and *A mellifera*).[17] As such, there currently are no treatment measures that have been tested against these mites and none is registered for usage against them. In the event that *Euvarroa* do make the transition to *A mellifera*, immediate access to remedial measures could spell the difference between a brief incursion and a costly, ongoing issue. Without registered treatment measures, control options currently used against *Varroa* likely would be considered. *Euvarroa* share an important common feature with *V destructor* in their lifecycle: a protracted dispersal stage. *Euvarroa* are able to spend substantially longer in this stage than *Varroa*.[25,26,51] This likely renders them vulnerable to many of the contact and fumigant insecticides currently registered for usage against *Varroa*.

Chemical control options against *Varroa* include[46]
  Synthetic miticides
  - Apistan (fluvalinate)
  - Apivar (amitraz)
  - CheckMite+ (coumaphos)
  - Essential oils:
    - ApiLifeVar (thymol, eucalyptol, menthol, and camphor)
    - Apiguard/Thymovar (thymol)
  Organic acids
  - Formic Pro/Mite Away Quick Strips (formic acid)
  - HopGuard II (hops beta acids)
  - Oxalic acid (oxalic acid dihydrate)
Cultural control options include
  Brood interruption
  Comb culling
  Drone brood removal
  Screened bottom/sticky board usage
  Thermal treatment
  Usage of resistant stock

Undoubtedly, some of these options would prove more effective than others against this parasite. Synthetic miticidal formulations like Amitraz, which has not proved effective against Tropi mites, would potentially be effective in managing *Euvarroa* in addition to the organic acid options.[37,46] Brood interruption, however, is unlikely to be an effective means of management. *Euvarroa* are well able to survive lengthy periods without brood available and appear to be unharmed by these protracted stretches without brood. If not coupled with a chemical treatment, this likely will do little else than slow the population growth of both the parasites and their host colony. Drone brood removal may prove effective if *Euvarroa* maintain a strong preference for drone brood, as is seen in *Varroa.*

Clinics Care Points

- *A mellifera* colonies found to be infested with *Euvarroa* should be reported to the governing biosecurity body in the region and the colony likely will be destroyed.
- *Euvarroa* appear very similar to the common *V destructor*; thus, suspect specimens should be delivered to an acarologist for final identification.

ASIAN HORNETS: *VESPA MANDARINIA* AND VESPA VELUTINA
Background

Within the wasp genus *Vespa* (hornets), multiple hornet species have developed a predatory association with honey bees.[52] None are better known for this behavior than *V mandarinia* (AGH) and the bee-hawking hornet *V velutina* (YLH). Recent incursions of both species in the west have promoted substantially greater interest in the biology and behavior of both species.[18,53] Both AGHs and YLHs are large wasps but YLHs are among the smallest of the *Vespa*, measuring between 17 mm and 22 mm. The AGH is better known for its size and its stout-bodied profile with workers, measuring 25 mm to 40 mm, and some queens reaching 50 mm in length.[11,54]

Vespa collect plant pulp within the environment and process it via maceration into a paper-like substance from which they construct their nests. In AGHs, nests consistently are constructed below ground in hollows left by partially unearthed trees or abandoned rodent burrows.[55,56] YLH nests typically are constructed in open-air suspended from tree branches or man-made structures.[57] The colony itself consist of 3 morphologically distinct castes (workers, queens, and drones). The best known of these are the workers because they are routinely active at a substantial distance from the colony itself.[52] Workers are the smallest of the 3 forms and are the foraging units of the colony. Their actions outside of the colony are limited to food and building resource procurement. Within the nest, they work to feed larvae, enlarge the cavity that the nest occupies, expand the size of the nest by constructing more paper cells, and maintaining the security of the nest via aggressive protective tactics.[11,52,54] In a mature nest, the queen never is seen outside of its confines but she is the most important hornet to target in management efforts.[52] Drones (male reproductives) can be a seasonal indicator of the presence of a colony but because they do not return to the nest after leaving, their capture is of limited utility.

Impact on Apis mellifera

Although human health impacts from *Vespa* stings certainly are cause for concern, the most pronounced and widespread impact likely would be to the industry of beekeeping.[55,58] Within their native range, AGHs and YLHs are blamed for the destruction of thousands of honey bee colonies annually.[11,59] Among honey bee species, *A mellifera* are uniquely vulnerable to the coordinated predation of *Vespa* species, showing little to no effective defense against these predators.[11,60] Just a few dozen AGHs can wipe out even the strongest *A mellifera* colony.[11]

AGHs and YLHs differ in their tactics. Although both conduct coordinated attacks on honey bee colonies, successful AGH raids invariably result in the death of the targeted colony. These raids start with a scout hornet locating a vulnerable honey bee colony. The scout returns to the colony with a squadron of sisters (approximately 2 or 3 dozen) that rapidly move through the colony aggressively decapitating every moving bee therein. Their focus is not the honey or pollen present in the colony but the heavily proteinaceous brood, which can fuel the growth of large numbers of their hungry drones and queens. Brood collection and relocation to the colony may take days because the hornets work to maximize exploitation of their prey.[11] It is during this time that beekeepers are most at risk because AGHs defend an occupied honey bee colony with all of the ferocity with which they would defend their own nest, potentially resulting in substantial injury or even death.[11,61,62]

YLHs by comparison do not invade honey bee colonies that they have targeted. They typically capture returning honey bee foragers at the colony's entrance. Such prey is caught on the wing in a behavior, known as *hawking*.[63,64] Hawking is common and honey bee colonies may survive a few bouts of such behavior; however, persistent hawking can lead to the decline and collapse of the colony, as has been noted throughout the introduced range of this hornet.[65] Honey bee colonies are at greatest risk of attack from both species in the fall when the protein demands of the colony trigger these predatory behaviors.[52] Unlike parasitic infestation or pathogenic infection, hornet attacks resulting in the death of a colony do not signal immediate threat to colonies nearby. A nest that has successfully extracted all of the protein it needs from a large honey bee colony has no need to coordinate strikes on nearby colonies to support the production of reproductives. After reproductives are produced, the colony declines and dies, ending the threat of further attacks for that season.[11,52] Thus, a single hornet's nest is unlikely to wipe out an entire apiary the way that a particularly virulent, highly transmissible infection can.

Detection/identification

Establishing live capture traps, baited with fruit juices and vinegar, in the environment can be effective in determining the density of these predators and can help locate a hornet nest.[11,66] Small GPS tracking devices can be fastened to captured worker hornets and upon their release, they can be followed back to the parent colony. These efforts are effective only when traps are monitored frequently. As such, outreach to organized public groups with a stake in whether this pest becomes established in the ecosystem can greatly increase the resolution of monitoring efforts. Specimens must be identified positively as female wasps of AGH or YLH prior to efforts to locate the colony to avoid wasting time and valuable resources. Once captured, AGHs can be distinguished easily from other wasps in North America by their large size alone. No social wasps in North America reach the same dimensions.[67,68] Attention to their ostentatious coloration can provide further confidence in a positive identification because the color morph detected so far in North America typically is bright orange with a striped abdomen alternating between bands of black and orange.[69]

The YLHs get their common name from the distinctively yellow tibia and tarsi of each leg. The nigrithorax color morph currently is the most broadly distributed geographically and is characterized by its dark brown to black thoracic region. Both the abdomen and head are dark brown to black as well but gradient to yellow toward the stinger on the abdomen and toward the mandibles on the head. In both species, drones have visibly longer antennae than female wasps and no stinger, but appear similar in most other regards.

Management

Successful protection of honey bee colonies from Asian hornets differs depending on the species of concern. Preventing an AGH scout from entering a honey bee colony typically prevents a coordinated raid on the colony thereby protecting it from the worst effects of this species.[11,70] Traps that allow only for the 1-way entry of hornets to a hollow chamber separate from the nest can be attached to the entrance of a honey bee colony. In Japan, these traps have been broadly effective at capturing dozens of hornets in a season. Colonies with these traps have shown full protection from hornet incursion with 0% losses compared with a 100% loss rate for colonies lacking traps in the same study.[70] By contrast, the bee-hawking behaviors of YLHs render such a system ineffective. YLHs are disinclined to enter honey bee colonies but 1-way traps with attractive baits (eg, apple juice and vinegar) suspended elsewhere in the environment have been used to mixed effect in some regions of expanded range of this insect.[18]

Of the potential long-term management options, population reduction via toxic bait has been the most effective on other related social wasp species.[71] These programs involve the deposition of poison-laced baits in areas of the environment where populations of the hornets are present or suspected to be present. Foraging worker hornets consume this bait and distribute the poison via trophallaxis ensuring that the reproductives of the colony also are impacted. Although these methods can destroy the entire parent colony by targeting the queen, there is substantial potential for nontarget impacts because these baits are nonspecific and attract a broad range of foraging animals.[18,71] Pilot efforts recently have been undertaken in China to dispatch hornet nests at high altitudes with the assistance of a flamethrower attached to a remotely controlled drone. Such methods may prove effective against open-air nesting species like YLHs but will not have an impact on subterranean species, such as AGHs.

Clinics Care Points

- Most important in managing the impact of AGHs on a colony is preventing the entrance of a foraging scout.
- Entrance reducers show some efficacy in preventing AGHs from gaining access but are ineffective in managing YLHs.
- Traps for live capture of Asian hornets must have a separate compartment from the bait or the hornets will likely drown or become covered in food debris, which may impede flight.
- Traps are best baited with a combination of fruit juice and fermented fluids, such as vinegar or alcohol.

CONCLUSION

It is not a given that these foreign honey bee pests will become an established threat in North America; however, history has shown that the wisest course of action is to be prepared. Spread into other countries often is the clearest indication that an organism is of heightened risk to spread further.[72] In addition to updating biosecurity regulations and documentation of the shifting taxonomic landscape, it is imperative to begin conducting research broadly on effective management and eradication tactics for high-risk organisms. Establishment of such pests would require adoption of management strategies uncommon in this region of the world. Research conducted in the native range of these pests or in areas where invasive populations have first emerged often are helpful in the early stages of drafting management protocols. Those studies are adapted, however, to the context in which they were conducted and can be tailored to ecosystems and a unique apicultural context. Establishing targeted studies of these foreign pests prior to their incursion in North America is critical to ongoing preparedness efforts.

DISCLOSURE STATEMENT

The author has nothing to disclose.

REFERENCES

1. Haldane JBS. Aristotle's account of bees''dances'. J Hellenic Stud 1955;75:24–5.
2. Bailey L, Ball B. Honey bee pathology. 2nd edition, 1991. p. 1-9.
3. Oldroyd BP, Nanork P. Conservation of Asian honey bees. Apidologie 2009;40(3): 296–312.
4. Lo N, Gloag RS, Anderson DL, et al. A molecular phylogeny of the genus Apis suggests that the Giant Honey Bee of the Philippines, A. breviligula Maa, and the Plains Honey Bee of southern India, A. indica Fabricius, are valid species. Syst Entomol 2010;35(2):226–33.
5. Oldroyd BP, Wongsiri S. Asian honey bees: biology, conservation, and human interactions. Harvard University Press; 2009.
6. Chantawannakul P, Ramsey S. The overview of honey bee diversity and health status in Asia. Asian beekeeping in the 21st century. Springer; 2018. p. 1–39.
7. Asia I. Food and agriculture organization of the United Nations 2013. FAO, Rome.
8. Khongphinitbunjong K, De Guzman LI, Burgett MD, et al. Behavioral responses underpinning resistance and susceptibility of honeybees to Tropilaelaps mercedesae. Apidologie 2012;43(5):590–9.
9. Beaurepaire AL, Truong TA, Fajardo AC, et al. Host specificity in the honeybee parasitic mite, Varroa spp. in Apis mellifera and Apis cerana. PloS one 2015; 10(8):e0135103.
10. Boot WJ, Tan NQ, Dien PC, et al. Reproductive success of Varroa jacobsoni in brood of its original host, Apis cerana, in comparison to that of its new host, A. mellifera (Hymenoptera: Apidae). Bull Entomol Res 1997;87(2):119–26.
11. Matsuura M, SAKAGAMI SF. A Bionomic Sketch of the Giant Hornet, Vespa mandarinia, a Serious Pest for Japanese Apiculture (With 12 Text-figures and 5 Tables). Jour Faa Sci Hokkaido Univ Ser Vi Zool 1973;19(1):125–62.
12. Paxton RJ, Klee J, Korpela S, et al. Nosema ceranae has infected Apis mellifera in Europe since at least 1998 and may be more virulent than Nosema apis. Apidologie 2007;38(6):558–65.
13. Chantawannakul P, De Guzman LI, Li J, et al. Parasites, pathogens, and pests of honeybees in Asia. Apidologie 2016;47(3):301–24.
14. Anderson DL, Roberts JM. Standard methods for Tropilaelaps mites research. J Apicultural Res 2013;52(4):1–16.
15. Roberts JM, Schouten CN, Sengere RW, et al. Effectiveness of control strategies for Varroa jacobsoni and Tropilaelaps mercedesae in Papua New Guinea. Exp Appl Acarol 2020;80(3):399–407.
16. Anderson D, Trueman J. Varroa jacobsoni (Acari: Varroidae) is more than one species. Exp Appl Acarol 2000;24(3):165–89.
17. Mossadegh M. Development ofEuvarroa sinhai (Acarina: Mesostigmata), a parasitic mite ofApis florea, onA. mellifera worker brood. Exp Appl Acarol 1990; 9(1–2):73–8.
18. Monceau K, Bonnard O, Thiéry D. Vespa velutina: a new invasive predator of honeybees in Europe. J Pest Sci 2014;87(1):1–16.

19. de Guzman L, Williams G, Khongphinitbunjong K, et al. Ecology, Life History, and Management of Tropilaelaps Mites. J Econ Entomol 2017;110(2):319.
20. Anderson DL, Morgan MJ. Genetic and morphological variation of bee-parasitic Tropilaelaps mites (Acari: Laelapidae): new and re-defined species. Exp Appl Acarol 2007;43(1):1–24.
21. Delfinado-Baker M, Baker E. A new species of Tropilaelaps parasitic on honey bees. Am Bee J 1982;122(6):416–7.
22. Chantawannakul P, Ramsey S, Khongphinitbunjong K, et al. Tropilaelaps mite: an emerging threat to European honey bee. Curr Opin Insect Sci 2018.
23. Khongphinitbunjong K, de Guzman LI, Buawangpong N, et al. Observations on the removal of brood inoculated with Tropilaelaps mercedesae (Acari: Laelapidae) and the mite's reproductive success in Apis mellifera colonies. Exp Appl Acarol 2014;62(1):47–55.
24. Phokasem P, de Guzman LI, Khongphinitbunjong K, et al. Feeding by Tropilaelaps mercedesae on pre-and post-capped brood increases damage to Apis mellifera colonies. Scientific Rep 2019;9(1):1–12.
25. Beetsma J, Boot WJ, Calis J. Invasion behaviour of Varroa jacobsoni Oud.: from bees into brood cells. Apidologie 1999;30(2–3):125–40.
26. Akratanakul P, Burgett M. Euvarroa sinhai Delfinado and Baker (Acarina: Mesostigmata): a parasitic mite of Apis florea. J Apicultural Res 1976;15(1):11–3.
27. Khan K. Beekeeping in Pakistan (history, potential, and current Status) 2020.
28. Woyke J. Further investigations into control of the parasite bee mite Tropilaelaps clareae without medication. J apicultural Res 1985;24(4):250–4.
29. Raffique MK, Mahmood R, Aslam M, et al. Control of Tropilaelaps clareae mite by using formic acid and thymol in honey bee Apis mellifera L. colonies. Pakistan J Zoolog 2012;44(4):1129–35.
30. Luo QH, Zhou T, Dai PL, et al. Prevalence, intensity and associated factor analysis of Tropilaelapsmercedesae infesting Apismellifera in China. Exp Appl Acarol 2011;55(2):135–46.
31. Griffiths DA. Functional morphology of the mouthparts of Varroa jacobsoni and Tropilaelaps clareae as a basis for the interpretation of their life-styles. Africanized honey bees and bee mites/editors, Glen R Needham[et al], Ellis Horwood Ltd, 1988.
32. Kanbar G, Engels W. Ultrastructure and bacterial infection of wounds in honey bee (Apis mellifera) pupae punctured by Varroa mites. Parasitol Res 2003;90(5):349–54.
33. Ramsey SD, Ochoa R, Bauchan G, et al. Varroa destructor feeds primarily on honey bee fat body tissue and not hemolymph. Proc Natl Acad Sci 2019;201818371.
34. Khongphinitbunjong K, De Guzman LI, Tarver MR, et al. Interactions of Tropilaelaps mercedesae, honey bee viruses and immune response in Apis mellifera. J Apicultural Res 2015;54(1):40–7.
35. Woyke J. Survival and prophylactic control of Tropilaelaps clareae infesting Apis mellifera colonies in Afghanistan. Apidologie 1984;15(4):421–34.
36. Gilbert C. Visual control of cursorial prey pursuit by tiger beetles (Cicindelidae). J Comp Physiol A 1997;181(3):217–30.
37. Pettis JS, Rose R, Chaimanee V. Chemical and cultural control of Tropilaelaps mercedesae mites in honeybee (Apis mellifera) colonies in Northern Thailand. PloS one 2017;12(11):e0188063.
38. Delfinado MD, Baker EW. Varroidae, a new family of mites on honey bees (Mesostigmata: Acarina). J Wash Acad Sci 1974;4–10.

39. Rosenkranz P, Aumeier P, Ziegelmann B. Biology and control of Varroa destructor. J invertebrate Pathol 2010;103:S96–119.
40. Baker RA. The parasitic mites of honeybees–past, present and future. 2010. 1(4):1–7.
41. Koca AÖ, Kandemir İ. Diversity and distribution of dwarf honeybees in Iran and their role in natural and agricultural systems. The future role of dwarf honey bees in natural and agricultural systems. CRC Press; 2020. p. 259–72.
42. de Guzman LI, Simone-Finstrom M, Cervancia C, et al. Tropilaelaps species identification and viral load evaluation of Tropilaelaps and Varroa mites and their Apis mellifera hosts in Palawan, Philippines. J Invertebr Pathol 2020;170:107324.
43. Koeniger N, Koeniger G, De Guzman L, et al. Survival of Euvarroa sinhai Delfinado and Baker (Acari, Varroidae) on workers of Apis cerana Fabr, Apis florea Fabr and Apis mellifera L in cages. Apidologie 1993;24(4):403–10.
44. Ramsey S, Gulbronson CJ, Mowery J, et al. A Multi-Microscopy Approach to Discover the Feeding Site and Host Tissue Consumed by Varroa destructor on Host Honey Bees. Microsc Microanal 2018;24(S1):1258–9.
45. Kitprasert C. Parasitism by the brood mite, Euvarroa sinhai Delfinado and Baker (Acari: Varroidae) on the dwarf honey bee, Apis florea F.(Hymenoptera: Apidae) in Thailand 1994.
46. Coalition HBH. Tools for Varroa management a guide to effective varroa sampling & control 2018. Available at: https://honeybeehealthcoalition.org/wp-content/uploads/2018/06/HBHC-Guide_Varroa_Interactive_7thEdition_June2018.pdf.
47. Fan Q-H, Parmar P, George S, et al. An improved technique for quantifying infestation level of external mites (Acari) on honey bees. J Apicultural Res 2018;57(2):317–20.
48. Lekprayoon C, Tangkanasing P. Euvarroa wongsirii, a new species of bee mite from Thailand. Int J 1991;17(4):255–8.
49. Delfinado-Baker M. Morphology and Developmental changes of Euvarroa sinhai Delfinado & baker (Acari: Varroidae) from the honeybee apis florea (Hymenoptera: Apidae). Int J 1987;13(3):203–8.
50. Morin CE, Otis GW. Observations on the morphology and biology of Euvarroa wongsirii (Mesostigmata: Varroidae), a parasite of Apis andreniformis (Hymenoptera: Apidae). Int J 1993;19(2):167–72.
51. Xie X, Huang ZY, Zeng Z. Why do Varroa mites prefer nurse bees? Scientific Rep 2016;6:28228.
52. Matsuura M, Yamane S. Biology of the vespine wasps. Springer Verlag; 1990.
53. Looney C, Spichiger S-E, Salp K, et al. Vespa mandarinia in the Pacific Northwest-Initial responses to an invasion by the world's largest hornet 2020. Available at: https://www.researchgate.net/publication/342610876_Vespa_mandarinia_in_the_Pacific_Northwest_-_Initial_responses_to_an_invasion_by_the_world%27s_largest_hornet.
54. Lee JX. Notes on Vespa analis and Vespa mandarinia (Hymenoptera, Vespidae) in Hong Kong, and a key to all Vespa species known from the SAR. Hong Kong Entomol Bull 2010;2(2):31–6.
55. MATSUURA M, KOIKE K. Studies on the ecology of social wasps and bees in urban environments 1. Records on aerial nests of the giant hornet, Vespa mandarinia japonica (Hymenoptera: Vespidae) within human buildings. Med Entomol Zoolog 2002;53(3):183–6.
56. Archer ME. Taxonomy, distribution and nesting biology of species of the genera Provespa Ashmead and Vespa Linnaeus (Hymenoptera, Vespidae). Entomologist''s Monthly Mag 2008;144(1727):69.

57. Franklin DN, Brown MA, Datta S, et al. Invasion dynamics of Asian hornet, Vespa velutina (Hymenoptera: Vespidae): a case study of a commune in south-west France. Appl Entomol Zoolog 2017;52(2):221–9.

58. Yanagawa Y, Morita K, Sugiura T, et al. Cutaneous hemorrhage or necrosis findings after Vespa mandarinia (wasp) stings may predict the occurrence of multiple organ injury: a case report and review of literature. Clin Toxicol 2007;45(7):803–7.

59. Shah F, Shah T. Vespa velutina, a serious pest of honey bees in Kashmir. Bee World 1991;72(4):161–4.

60. McClenaghan B, Schlaf M, Geddes M, et al. Behavioral responses of honey bees, Apis cerana and Apis mellifera, to Vespa mandarinia marking and alarm pheromones. J Apicultural Res 2019;58(1):141–8.

61. Liu Z, Li X-D, Guo B-H, et al. Acute interstitial nephritis, toxic hepatitis and toxic myocarditis following multiple Asian giant hornet stings in Shaanxi Province, China. Environ Health Prev Med 2016;21(4):231–6.

62. Hirano K, Tanikawa A. Ocular injury caused by the sprayed venom of the Asian giant hornet (Vespa mandarinia). Case Rep Ophthalmol 2020;11(2):430–5.

63. Tan K, Radloff S, Li J, et al. Bee-hawking by the wasp, Vespa velutina, on the honeybees Apis cerana and A. mellifera. Naturwissenschaften 2007;94(6):469–72.

64. Villemant C, Barbet-Massin M, Perrard A, et al. Predicting the invasion risk by the alien bee-hawking Yellow-legged hornet Vespa velutina nigrithorax across Europe and other continents with niche models. Biol Conserv 2011;144(9):2142–50.

65. Laurino D, Lioy S, Carisio L, et al. Vespa velutina: An Alien Driver of Honey Bee Colony Losses. Diversity 2020;12(1):5.

66. Lebrun A. Asian giant hornet control program in Washington state. Available at: https://www.aphis.usda.gov/plant_health/ea/downloads/2020/ea-agh-draft.pdf.

67. Kimsey L, Carpenter J. The Vespinae of North America (Vespidae, Hymenoptera). J Hymenoptera Res 2012;28:37.

68. Shaw F, Weidhaas J Jr. Distribution and habits of the giant hornet in North America. J Econ Entomol 1956;49(2):275.

69. Smith-Pardo AH, Carpenter JM, Kimsey L. The diversity of hornets in the genus Vespa (Hymenoptera: Vespidae; Vespinae), their importance and interceptions in the United States. Insect Syst Divers 2020;4(3):2.

70. Matsuura M. Ecological study on vespine wasps (Hymenoptera: Vespidae) attacking honeybee colonies: I. seasonal changes in the frequency of visits to apiaries by vespine wasps and damage inflicted, especially in the absence of artificial protection. Appl Entomol Zoolog 1988;23(4):428–40.

71. Beggs JR, Brockerhoff EG, Corley JC, et al. Ecological effects and management of invasive alien Vespidae. BioControl 2011;56(4):505–26.

72. Lockwood JL, Hoopes MF, Marchetti MP. Invasion ecology. John Wiley & Sons; 2013.

Honey Bees
Disaster Preparedness and Response

Cynthia M. Faux, DVM, PhD, DACVIM-LA[a],*, Terry Ryan Kane, DVM, MS[b]

KEYWORDS

- Disaster • Planning and preparedness • Mitigation • Insurance • Honey bees

KEY POINTS

- Planning and mitigation can help minimize losses during a disaster.
- Identification of hazards/risks can aid in apiary location planning.
- Insurance programs can include honey bee businesses.

INTRODUCTION

A disaster can be a natural catastrophe, the result of a technological accident, or a human-caused event that results in severe property damage, deaths, and/or injuries. Because agriculture relies on weather, climate, and water availability, it is susceptible to multiple natural disasters. Global climate change is contributing to weather extremes: intense rainstorms, tornadoes, hurricanes, flooding, and mudslides.[1] This last decade has been one of the hottest on record, bringing prolonged and dangerous droughts and wildfires, jeopardizing human and animal food supplies.[2] Technical accidents affecting farms and apiaries can be the result of industrial accidents, chemical spills, pesticide (mis)applications, and transportation or warehousing mishaps. Beekeepers have experienced introduced pests, such as varroa (*Varroa destructor*), tracheal mites (*Acarapis woodi*), and small hive beetles (*Aethina tumida*). We must be vigilant to avoid future introductions and spread of the Asian Giant hornet (*Vespa mandarinia*) or Tropi mites (*Tropilaelaps* spp.) and the associated sequela.

DISCUSSION

Disasters can be widespread or local. Local, or personal, disasters would include such events as vandalism, toxic spills, bears, local weather events, and structure fires. More widespread disasters would include wildfires, hurricanes, flooding, and other major weather events. For beekeepers, a disaster can be a personal loss of great significance that is a stand-alone event or is part of a larger enveloping regional disaster.

[a] Veterinary Medicine, The University of Arizona College of Veterinary Medicine, 1580 E Hanley Boulevard, PO Box 210506, Oro Valley, AZ 85737, USA; [b] A2 Bee Vet, Ann Arbor, MI 48103, USA
* Corresponding author.
E-mail address: cfaux@arizona.edu

Vet Clin Food Anim 37 (2021) 559–567
https://doi.org/10.1016/j.cvfa.2021.06.015
0749-0720/21/© 2021 Elsevier Inc. All rights reserved.

The significant loss of bees, colonies, equipment, and even entire apiaries can be personally and financially catastrophic. Veterinarians can assist apiarists in developing resiliency against potential disasters. Disaster planning is a field with excellent resources available to veterinarians to help apiarists plan for the worst. These resources include www.ready.gov, https://emergency.cdc.gov/, and https://www.avma.org/resources-tools/animal-health-and-welfare/disaster-preparedness.

Before any continuity of business disaster planning can occur, however, personal safety and family disaster planning must take priority. No one can effectively respond to a disaster situation if they are concerned for the safety of themselves and their family. Excellent personal and household disaster planning information is available at the following sites: https://ready.gov, https://www.avma.org/resources-tools/animal-health-and-welfare/disaster-preparedness to assist the apiarist (and veterinarian) in disaster planning for their household.

Planning

Several components must be incorporated into a disaster plan, whether personal or business. The first component is the recognition of the potential risks. For example, inhabitants of Washington State have little concern for hurricanes, whereas those in Florida should not be concerned with volcanic eruptions as an immediate potential threat. The potential for impact by wildfires, floods, earthquakes, and so forth will play a role in determining apiary placement, as will more localized hazards, such as the presence of bears, neighbors, sprayed fields, or roads.

In addition to identifying hazards and risks, planning includes determining the vulnerabilities of the honey bees to the hazard and establishing the potential consequences. For example, if the hazard is flooding and the apiary is located on high ground and therefore not vulnerable, a flood would have little immediate consequence to the hives. However, if the apiary is located on a portion of a flood plain and flooding would potentially wipe out any colonies located in that site, the consequences and losses would be high (**Fig. 1**). In addition, although the physical hives may be safe from a flood, widespread damage to the fields and plants in the area may create an instant nectar dearth and necessitate supplemental feeding of the colonies.

Numerous factors play a role in the vulnerability of a site to disasters. Factors may include road access (can the apiarist quickly respond to a threat by moving the hives) and access to resources to move the hives (trucks, personnel, time). Vulnerabilities

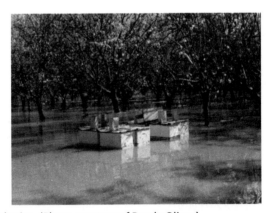

Fig. 1. Flooded colonies. (*Photo courtesy of* Randy Oliver.)

also include lack of financial resources to accomplish a move and the existence of a secondary safe site.

The consequences of a loss may not be limited to the loss of the impacted bees and equipment hardware, but may include other valuables, such as the loss of honey and other saleable products, unique genetics, the pollination income from the loss of the crop, and the permanent loss of clients (future pollination income) who were irreparably harmed by a disaster event.

An analysis of the hazards, vulnerabilities, and consequences will allow the veterinarian and apiarist to determine the risk analysis for the site. Following a risk analysis, determining what resources may be available in the event of a tragedy yields the beginnings of a strategic plan.

Planning an apiary site also includes the protection of neighbors, pets, innocent passers-by, and livestock. Environmental hazards can prove dangerous to the beekeeper as well as hives, such as large broken branches or a toppling tree (**Fig. 2**). Local and state ordinances and laws can impact where an apiary may be established, particularly in urban and suburban regions. Hive registration is required in many states and jurisdictions. Some states offer limited liability protection to apiarists who follow state and local laws regarding beekeeping. Thus, familiarity with the state regulations and local ordinances regarding beekeeping can be useful for the beekeeper and veterinarian.

Mitigation

The purpose of mitigation is to lessen the risk of a disaster impact. For example, if there are no reasonable alternatives to placing an apiary in a flood-prone site, one may choose to place hives on taller stands, provide a top hive entrance in case the regular entrance is submerged, or develop a plan to move the hives if threatened by flood. For pollination services, the location of the hives in relevance to the crops being pollinated requires attention to detail regarding the potential risks to the bees and equipment. For stable apiaries, long-term sustainability also requires such attention. Mitigation strategies also include placing vulnerable genetics in multiple locations, preferably ones with less likelihood of impact. Ensuring adequate resources are available for evacuation, as well as flexibility in hive design or location may also serve to mitigate risk.

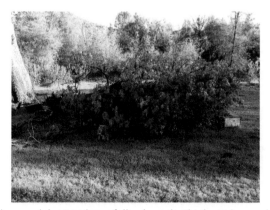

Fig. 2. Nuc hives damaged due to a large fallen branch. This branch was also a hazard to any apiarist working with the hives. (*Photo courtesy of* Randy Oliver.)

Bear mitigation is a common practice in regions with established bear populations. Bears can cause a tremendous amount of damage to hives by destroying woodenware while consuming brood and honey (**Fig. 3**). An apiary is an appealing target, and bears may frequent it as an easy feeding ground. Electric fencing can provide protection to apiaries, but ideally should be installed in advance of bear predation.

Theft and vandalism are, unfortunately, concerns. Identification of the hive boxes, such as branding, displaying painting with owner information, and/or inserting microchips in boxes may help deter theft and aid in the recovery of stolen equipment. Installing camera monitoring equipment in the apiary can provide information to law enforcement.

Fire mitigation includes careful handling of lit smokers to avoid setting grass or brush ablaze and also extends to care in parking over tall, dry, grassy areas where hot portions of the exhaust/engine could initiate a fire. One may choose to carry a fire extinguisher in the vehicle or have one nearby while working a colony. Fire risk assessment may suggest clearing of grass, brush, and trees around the apiary to help mitigate the impact of a large-scale wildfire (**Fig. 4**).

Biosecurity is an important mitigation strategy in preventing disease from entering the apiary and in preventing the spreading of disease from one colony or apiary to another. Veterinarians have extensive training in biosecurity and can help identify areas for improvement in the apiarist's routine hive inspection practices. Biosecurity includes cleaning and disinfecting hive tools and gloves, awareness and identification of diseased colonies, and working with potentially diseased or weak colonies after healthy colonies have been examined. Careful inspection before sharing frames of brood or honey between colonies can help mitigate the spread of disease from one colony to another. Hive destruction may be required in some jurisdictions for American foulbrood diseased colonies and can result in significant financial consequences.

Direct pesticide application to fields with foraging bees, as well as pesticide drift to nontarget fields are distinct hazards. Such pesticide disasters can be mitigated by joining organizations such as Fieldwatch.com, a national collaboration among farmers, beekeepers, and professional pesticide applicators. This tool has been designed to improve communication between applicators and beekeepers and has been shown to be very effective in protecting honey-producing colonies, as well as other pollinators, from sprayed pesticide application in participating states.

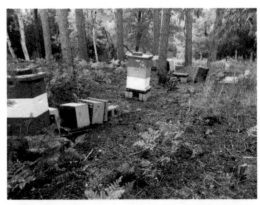

Fig. 3. An example of bear destruction in an apiary. Strewn boxes and frames litter the site. Hives still standing are at risk when the perpetrator invariably returns. (*Photo courtesy of* Ana Heck.)

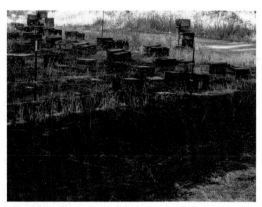

Fig. 4. Hives burned from a wildfire. (*Photo courtesy of* Randy Oliver.)

Veterinarians can encourage communication with neighbors regarding the danger of pesticides to bees, particularly in urban and suburban areas. The sensitivity of pollinators to chemicals applied to lawns and ornamental plants may not be common knowledge. The placement of signage (such as Do Not Spray) on the property may be useful in situations where a local jurisdiction sprays for weeds in ditches and roadsides. "Opt-out" programs may exist in local jurisdictions that allow individual producers to avoid having herbicides applied to their property. Contacting those entities that may spray (eg, county highway department, power company) may provide solutions to prevent inadvertent intoxication of the apiary.

Response Phase

Planning and mitigation strategies can only go so far, and it may be necessary to respond to a disaster. Each disaster is unique and may vary in scope from isolated management by the beekeeper to more complex situations that require coordination with local authorities, particularly in the case of multi-agency responses to wildfires, hurricanes, tornadoes, and floods. Apiary evacuation may not be an option if human life is endangered or if the hazard is fast moving (eg, wildfires, tornadoes). If evacuation is an option, there are a number of questions that need to be considered. Are the necessary resources (eg, people, equipment, vehicles) available? Is the evacuation route safe and the destination out of danger? Can the hives be safely secured while en route? Are health or transport certificates required for a destination in another state?

Bees may not be welcome at livestock evacuation centers. However, local response agencies may be able to assist in identifying secure temporary locations for hives. As honey bees are considered livestock, bee incidents requiring a coordinated response are often managed by the state agricultural authority/agency. Other resources include the state Extension agency and university entomology departments.

U.S. Beekeeper Profit Protections in Case of Disasters

Beekeeping is a significant niche commodity in agriculture, contributing billions of dollars in pollination services as well as hive products. There are a number of insurance products, both federal and private, to help beekeepers mitigate losses.

Federal Insurance Programs

Federal Crop Insurance now includes apiculture, is subsidized, and prices are set and managed by the US Department of Agriculture (USDA)-RMA (Risk Management

Agency). Thus, regardless from whom the farmer buys insurance, the rates will be the same. Farmers are expected to apply good apiary practices, as well as keep detailed records of production by location. The Federal Crop Insurance Programs only cover honey bees used for pollination, breeding, or honey production. They do not cover other bees, such as leaf cutter bees, mason bees, or feral bees. To be eligible for coverage, the farmer/apiarist must own or rent the farm with at least a 10% interest. For a premium subsidy, the farmer/apiarist must have an AD-1026 on file with the Farm Services Agency (FSA) office before billing. This form, the Highly Erodible Land Conservation and Wetland Conservation Certification was mandated in the 2014 Farm Bill and links conservation compliance with eligibility for premium support paid under federal crop insurance programs. Otherwise, the farmer will have to pay full price for their premiums. Information such as what varroa management practices are used, honey sales figures, and equipment expenses should be tracked. For some programs, good records of purchases, sales, production, and treatments are required to document losses when filing a claim. Fair market values for colonies vary by year and are state/county specific. Always consult a Crop Insurance Agent for program requirements, benefits, and costs. The Web site for an agent locator is https://www.rma.usda.gov/informationtools/agentlocator.

There are a number of federal crop insurance policies that cover honey bees. These federal policies are subsidized, and prices are set and managed by the USDA-RMA and purchased through qualified independent insurance agencies:

Whole Farm Revenue Protection (WFRP)[3] is the first established subsidized federal crop insurance policy available to farmers nationwide. This policy provides a safety net for all commodities on the farm, including honey bees, under one insurance policy. WFRP provides protection against lost revenue due to production and market price risks from unavoidable natural causes. The more diverse the operation, the more crops that are grown, or the more diverse products sold, the lower the premium rate. Records must show revenue and a producer must have 5 years of tax history from farming (or 3 for a new farmer and/or a qualified veteran farmer/rancher). This insurance is considered an umbrella farm policy for any cause of loss. There is a cap of $2 million USD for animal crops, but can be up to $8.5 million USD with other additional crops.

Apiculture Rainfall Index (API)[4] is an insurance product based on low precipitation, not production/loss. Apiculture is practiced in diverse areas with varying climate conditions and seasonal forage crops, so lower than average rainfall could affect honey production. This insurance product was designed to cover the precipitation patterns in different regions of the country. API is the most popular product for commercial operators, the rates are relatively low, and is effective in any state (most claims are in the western and high plains, the drought-prone states). The USDA-RMA sets a value on the hives and hive products as it relates to a rainfall index for the property's specific grid area over a discrete time period. The rainfall index uses the National Oceanic and Atmospheric Administration (NOAA) data using a grid system, and colonies are assigned to one or more grids. Payments and coverage are based on this grid system, where grids cover an area of 0.25° latitude by 0.25° longitude (roughly 17 miles × 17 miles at the equator). Rainfall index values are calculated by a weighted average of nearby NOAA weather stations and are reported in relation to historical average rainfall in that grid. Qualified agents can access historical rainfall data for specific regions. As with the other federal policies, the farmer must own, rent, or have written permission to be on the land to receive compensation.

Noninsured Crop Disaster Assistance Program (NAP)[5] covers production losses due to natural events (eg, damaging weather, floods, drought, earthquakes, or wildfires). This product is meant to help with catastrophic events affecting honey production, so even smaller producers can benefit from this protection. Diseases are also covered by the NAP; however, the producer must show that good farming practices were used to control/treat the disease(s). All honey is considered a single crop; this insurance is catastrophic coverage for honey production based on average hive production. Catastrophic coverage is 50% production at 55% of established market price with additional options at higher premiums. This insurance product is administered by USDA- FSA. This is not bought from an independent insurance agency but through the FSA. Crops and hives can be certified with the FSA.

Emergency Assistance for Livestock (ELAP)[6] for livestock, honey bees, and farm-raised fish. This program covers colony and hive losses, especially for overwintering problems like extreme cold and storms, and insures for any losses over a certain level. The "normal" expected hive mortality is established annually. For 2020, 22% was considered a normal/expected background mortality rate for an apiary, so only losses of more than 22% were considered for assistance. Hives must be certified with the FSA and there is no cost for timely certification. ELAP does cover structural damage, but damage from wildlife (such as bears) is not part of this coverage. Always consult a qualified USDA-FSA ELAP technician for qualified losses and reporting requirements in your county. As with NAP, this program is administered and purchased through the FSA.

Multi-Peril Crop Insurance (MPCI)[7] plans cover acts of nature as well as natural price losses. The MPCI is federally supported and regulated and is sold and serviced by private-sector crop insurance companies. Both the cost of insurance and the amount an insurer will pay for losses are tied to the value of the specific crop. MPCI is available for more than 120 different crops, although not all crops are covered in every geographic area. These policies must be purchased each growing season by deadlines established by the federal government, and before a crop is planted. If damage occurs early enough in the growing season, the policy may include incentives to replant, or penalties for not doing so. Many farmers purchase this product and rates are set for the county in which the apiarist farms. There are application and reporting requirements; keeping detailed records is important.

It is important to note that all federal programs have very strict deadlines/rules on timing and premium payments. It is highly recommended that producers consult a qualified agent up to a year before they want coverage. As with other insurance programs, there are discounts for purchasing multiple policies. A farmer can purchase API and WFRP at the same time and receive a discount toward the WFRP for having API (WFRP can get discounted due to the farmer having other RMA crop insurance products that protect a portion of the liability). The NAP does not discount WFRP, but a farmer should consult an agent regarding WFRP/NAP, as there are other important and notable interactions between the 2 programs. A qualified agent can make this process much easier.

Nonfederal Programs

Private safety-net options are also available to beekeepers. General liability coverage from the private sector is administered by insurance companies that specialize in farm liability. There are programs that will insure general farm liability for migratory, pollination, and other bee types (such as mason bees and alfalfa bees) raised by a business/farm. Veterinarians who work with apiarists should be aware of apiculture insurance programs available in their state to better advise and protect their clients from unforeseen disasters. Apiarists/farmers can ask their insurance agent if they are familiar with apiary crop insurance options and certified to sell the coverage needed. Special programs for beginning farmers, veterans, and socially disadvantaged/low-income farmers exist. These reduced-price programs are usually limited to 5 years.

Canadian Beekeeper Profit Protection

Six provinces of Canada's 10 provinces and 3 territories contain more than 70% of the country's beekeepers/colonies.[8] Canadian programs, titled AgriStability, are similar to the USDA's WFRP.[9] Canadian programs are cost shared between the provinces and the federal government of Canada, usually on a 60% federal and 40% provincial weighting depending on the program specifics. Programs are adjusted for specific losses/disasters. AgriInsurance (commonly known as crop insurance), is the first line of defense in Canada's system of business risk management. Each province has either a Crown Corporation or a branch of the provincial agriculture department responsible for administering the AgriInsurance programs.[10] The federal government's role is to provide program oversight by ensuring that the obligations under the Farm Income Protection Act, the Canada Production Insurance Regulations, and the Federal-Provincial-Territorial Framework Agreement (currently the Canadian Agricultural Partnership) are respected.

Canadian veterinarians can encourage beekeepers to contact their province for information on pollination protection plans, crop protection programs, and wildlife and environmental protection. Currently, 5 provinces offer insurance on bee mortality and overwintering protection. Bee mortality can have multiple causes; however, this plan only covers adverse weather, diseases, and/or pest infestations. To receive compensation, beekeepers are required to adhere to sound management practices to mitigate potential losses. Honey insurance is available in 4 provinces.

The prairie provinces of Alberta, Saskatchewan, and Manitoba are the major honey producers of Canada, whereas Eastern Canada and British Columbia commercial beekeepers provide the bulk of pollination services for specialty crops, particularly apples and blueberries.[11] Similar to almond crops in the United States, canola is a multibillion-dollar crop in Canada and half of the national bee herd is contracted to pollinate approximately 20 million acres of farmland in the western provinces of Alberta, Saskatchewan, and Manitoba.[11]

Wildlife (bears and ungulates) present greater challenges to hives in the north where these animals are more numerous, and most provinces offer a unique compensation program to pay for honey bee losses from bears. The program may also provide a first-time bear fencing subsidy.[12] Because Canada requires beehives to be registered, beekeepers may require an inspection to file a claim. The shorter growing seasons, harsh winter weather, and wildlife issues have made cold storage (overwintering indoors) increase in popularity, as it is in the United States, with commercial beekeepers.

CLINICS CARE POINTS

- Veterinarians can help their beekeeping clients with an evaluation of the hazards, vulnerabilities, and consequences to determine a risk analysis for the apiary site.
- Veterinarians can emphasize good biosecurity practices to prevent introduction of damaging honey bee pests to the apiary.
- Familiarization with insurance and indemnity programs available to producers in your area can help get impacted apiarists back into production.

ACKNOWLEDGMENTS

The authors thank Phillip Preston, Crop Insurance Specialist, GreenStone Farm Credit Services, Grand Rapids, MI, for his assistance in identifying and clarifying insurance programs in the United States that include honey bees (Phillip.Preston@ greenstonefcs.com).

DISCLOSURE

The authors have nothing to disclose.

REFERENCES

1. Climate.. Available at: https://www.noaa.gov/climate. Accessed March 21, 2021.
2. Brown K, editor. Hottest years on record. 2021. Available at: https://www.nasa. gov/press-release/2020-tied-for-warmest-year-on-record-nasa-analysis-shows. Accessed March 21, 2021.
3. Whole farm revenue protection. Available at: https://www.rma.usda.gov/en/Fact-Sheets/National-Fact-Sheets/Whole-Farm-Revenue-Protection-2020. Accessed March 21, 2021.
4. Apiculture pilot insurance program. Available at: https://www.rma.usda.gov/en/ Fact-Sheets/National-Fact-Sheets/Apiculture-Pilot-2017. Accessed March 21, 2021.
5. Noninsured Crop Disaster Assistance Program. Available at:https://www.fsa.usda. gov/Assets/USDA-FSA-Public/usdafiles/FactSheets/noninsured_crop_disaster_ assistance_program-nap-fact_sheet.pdf. https://www.fsa.usda.gov/Assets/USDA-FSA-Public/usdafiles/FactSheets/noninsured_crop_disaster_assistance_program-nap-fact_sheet.pdf. https://www.fsa.usda.gov/Assets/USDA-FSA-Public/usdafiles/ FactSheets/elap-general-2020-fact-sheet-1.pdf. Accessed March 21, 2021.
6. Emergency Assistance for Livestock, Honeybees and Farm-Raised Fish Program (ELAP). Available at: https://www.fsa.usda.gov/Assets/USDA-FSA-Public/usdafiles/ FactSheets/elap-honeybee-2020-fact-sheet.pdf. Accessed March 21, 2021.
7. Multiple peril crop insurance. 2020. Available at: https://content.naic.org/cipr_ topics/topic_crop_insurance.htm; https://content.naic.org/cipr_topics/topic_ crop_insurance.htm. Accessed March 21, 2021.
8. Statistical Overview of the Canadian Honey and Bee Industry, 2019. 2020. Available at: https://www.agr.gc.ca/eng/horticulture/horticulture-sector-reports/statistical-overview-of-the-canadian-honey-and-bee-industry-2019/?id=1594646761058#1. 1. Accessed March 21, 2021.
9. Agristability. 2020. Available at: https://www.agr.gc.ca/eng/agricultural-programs-and-services/agristability/?id=1291990433266%20Update. Accessed March 21, 2021.
10. Agrinsurance. 2019. Available at: https://www.agr.gc.ca/eng/agricultural-programs-and-services/agriinsurance-program/?id=1284665357886. Accessed March 21, 2021.
11. Available at:https://honeycouncil.ca/archive/honey_industry_overview.php#: %7E:text=The%20prairie%20provinces%20of%20Alberta,beekeeper%20with %20average%202%2C000%20colonies. Accessed March 21, 2021.
12. Honey Bee Wildlife Compensation Program. Available at: https://www.scic.ca/ wildlife/honey-bee-wildlife-compensation-program/. Accessed March 21, 2021.

Honey Bees and Humane Euthanasia

Britteny Kyle, DVM[a,b,*], Jeffrey R. Applegate Jr, DVM, DACZM[b,c,d]

KEYWORDS

- Euthanasia • Honey bees • Colony depopulation • Colony destruction

KEY POINTS

- Current methods of euthanasia of managed hive colonies vary from source to source regarding technique, materials, volume of agent used, and timing.
- There is a lack of guidelines and standards specific to the humane euthanasia of honey bees.
- Veterinarians working with honey bees must familiarize themselves with local, state/provincial, and federal rules and regulations regarding honey bee disease management and control.
- Veterinarians should approach euthanasia of honey bee colonies with the same professionalism and compassion as would be given to any other animal species.

INTRODUCTION

Euthanasia, or the provision of a good death, is a responsibility that veterinarians undertake for all animal species under their care.[1,2] Acceptable methods of euthanasia are species-specific and must ensure a rapid and irreversible loss of consciousness and be done in a manner that will reduce or eliminate pain and distress as much as possible.[1-3] Other factors that influence the appropriateness of the method include safety considerations for the operator and observers, economics of the procedure, and the aesthetics of the death itself.[2]

Performing humane euthanasia must also take into account how the animal is handled, especially up to the point of death, as well as the aftercare and disposal of the remains.[3] One must also consider the effect that the act of euthanasia may have on those observing as well as the environment in which the act is performed.[3]

As veterinarians become involved in honey bee health, there may be times that veterinarians are called on to advise on or perform euthanasia of a honey bee colony. It is

[a] Department of Population Medicine, Ontario Veterinary College, University of Guelph, 50 Stone Road East, Guelph, Ontario N1G 2W1, Canada; [b] Honey Bee Veterinary Consortium; [c] Nautilus Avian and Exotics Veterinary Specialists, 1010 Falkenberg Road, Brick, NJ 08724, USA; [d] Department of Clinical Sciences, North Carolina State University, College of Veterinary Medicine
* Corresponding author.
E-mail address: kyleb@uoguelph.ca

Vet Clin Food Anim 37 (2021) 569–575
https://doi.org/10.1016/j.cvfa.2021.06.011
vetfood.theclinics.com

expected that veterinarians approach honey bee euthanasia with the same level of professionalism and ethical standards as for any other animal species.

CURRENT METHODS OF DISPATCH AND EUTHANASIA OF HONEY BEES IN APICULTURE

Various methods have been used to dispatch, destroy, or euthanize honey bees and their associated colonies in the apicultural setting. Current methods of euthanasia of managed hive colonies vary from source to source with regards to technique, materials, volume of agent used, and timing. The Ontario Ministry of Agriculture, Food, and Rural Affairs (OMAFRA) describes in detail how to dispatch a hive using diesel fuel[4]; reminding you to collect the appropriate fire permits, if burning thereafter is necessary. The described method involves choosing a time when foragers will be contained within the hive and then sprinkling diesel fuel over the cluster of bees. The volume varies with the size of the hive, with 300-500 milliliters being recommended for a hive that is composed of one to two boxes and one liter for hives that are three to four boxes high. In hives with multiple boxes, the hive may need to be opened up in order to sufficiently douse the bees with the fuel, only using enough fuel to wet the bees as the fuel is not required as an accelerant. Following administration of the diesel fuel, the hive should be completely closed up for at least 10 minutes. After the waiting period, the adult bees should be checked to ensure they are immobilized; if any bees are still moving, more diesel fuel can be added to wet the still-alive bees".[4]

This method is also recommended in the US Department of Agriculture–Animal and Plant Health Inspection Service National Veterinary Accreditation Program training module #30: The Role of Veterinarians in Honey Bee Health.[5] Similar recommendations are found for New Zealand beekeepers, though, promoting petrol (gasoline) at similar volumes as that promoted by OMAFRA.[6] BeeAware, in Australia, similarly promotes petrol providing the specifics of "keep clear of the smoker" and defines a volume for use as 1 cup and repeat if bees remain alive.[7] An alternative option of dousing with soapy water is mentioned, but describes the likelihood of some bees escaping to other hives. In France, Dr. Vidal-Naquet[8] states that destruction of the colony is performed by asphyxiating the bees with a sulfur wick placed at the hive entrance and leaving the hive closed for about 15 minutes.

Extension sources in the United States recommend that, if desired, honey bees can be killed before burning (in cases of American foulbrood [AFB]) and that it should be completed quickly and safely.[9] In describing burning bees and equipment to eradicate AFB, the bees should be killed in the evening after all foraging activities have ceased. The method of killing described from this source is diesel fuel: 1 cup/hive body followed by a waiting period of 10 minutes for effect.[10]

Beekeepers may have their own methods of honey bee colony dispatch. An awareness of less traditional methods of "at-home euthanasia" of honey bees may be helpful when discussing and planning euthanasia protocols. Various blog sites recommend carbon dioxide (CO_2) via dry ice, which results in the bees "falling asleep" and expiring because of oxygen displacement by CO_2 as it fills the hive.[11] For this method to be effective, the hive must be well sealed, and it is understood that the dry ice is set on the frame top bars. Another blog-site suggestion was the use of CO_2 via paintball canisters delivered by a remote line obtained through a recreational sports shop. This method may require some skill and know-how, as pressurized gasses are being manipulated. Personal risk of freeze injury from chamber decompression is mentioned, but curiously, the explosive forces are not addressed.

Further suggestions found on blog conversations included adding sulfur-based fungicidal powder (90% sulfur) intended for plants to the smoker to kill the bees with sulfur-based smoke. A complication reported was that it took over an hour of smoking to kill the bees. Unfortunately, there was no discussion of the human health hazards nor potential environmental concerns.[12] Other anecdotal killing methods include stuffing the entrance with a gasoline-soaked rag or, similar to above, pouring gasoline in the hive (warning of explosive effects if set fire before fume dissipation), administration of liquid nitrogen to the hive (human health risk and availability concerns), dousing with rubbing alcohol, and closing the entrance followed by spraying the hive with diatomaceous earth.

In addition to managed hive euthanasia, relocation or eradication of feral colonies often comes into question. As with suggestions above, various options are found for accomplishing this task. Basic Internet searches discuss methods of relocating feral colonies versus killing the honey bees as though they were common pests. Humane relocation of feral populations is often accomplished by an educated, trained beekeeper or company. Suggestions of ridding feral bees in nonfarm situations by killing them include various methods, such as application of noxious pesticides or soapy water, that is, "If the nest is small and outside your home, you can try to destroy it using a solution of soapy water (one part liquid dish soap to four parts water) in a plastic spray bottle or garden sprayer."[13,14] Although feral colony management does not relate directly to euthanasia of kept hive colonies, it does allow for public education should a local honey bee veterinarian get a call about a feral colony.

DISCUSSION

There are several situations in which euthanasia of a honey bee colony may be recommended. The American Veterinary Medical Association (AVMA) *Guidelines for the Euthanasia of Animals: 2020 Edition* discusses honey bees, but only in so much as to mention that they are included as an invertebrate taxa that may have well-developed brains and/or complex behaviors with the ability to respond to noxious stimuli.[3] However, no further discussion of euthanasia or humane dispatch of a hive is covered in the text.[3] As with all animal species, euthanasia may be the best option to prevent prolonged and unnecessary suffering.[2,3] When a colony is not likely to improve with intervention or over time, euthanasia should be considered. Furthermore, veterinarians do not currently have many tools for supportive care and analgesia in honey bees that are often used to improve quality of life in other species. There also are no criteria for evaluation of pain, suffering, and welfare in colonies. Therefore, veterinarians should be proactive in making end-of-life decisions when conditions within the colony are likely terminal.

Although veterinarians must consider the welfare and best interest of the colony, other mitigating factors that can influence the decision for euthanasia include productivity, the economics of interventions, concern for other nearby colonies, and the prevention of transmissible disease. There are also times when the decision to euthanize may be mandated by local, provincial/state, or federal regulations and legislation. This occurrence is particularly true with the diagnosis of AFB, where many states and provinces have specific requirements in place under the Apiary Inspection Program. Euthanasia and destruction may also be required upon confirmation of foreign pests and diseases.

Veterinarians are encouraged to develop plans for honey bee euthanasia in advance. This plan will include consideration of the following[1]:

- How to recognize a sick colony

- Understanding when the appropriate authorities need to be alerted, as is often the case with AFB, and foreign pests and diseases
- The development of clinical endpoint criteria
- The method of euthanasia

Plans should also be discussed in advance with beekeepers with a valid veterinary-client-patient relationship if they are regularly using veterinary services in their operations.[2] Advance discussion will assist both veterinarians and beekeepers in making timely and appropriate end-of-life decisions. Veterinarians should recognize that beekeepers, or employees, may choose to perform euthanasia themselves. In this instance, veterinarians trained in honey bee health can still discuss and advise on euthanasia, and this could be incorporated into colony health management visits.[2]

A critical component of humane euthanasia is that it must be carried out in a way to reduce or eliminate distress in the animal.[1,3] Honey bees should be minimally handled before and during euthanasia. When possible, movement of colonies should be avoided until after euthanasia is complete. Euthanasia ideally should be performed at the end of the day to allow for the return of foragers and should occur within the hive. Veterinarians performing euthanasia should be confident in their ability to recognize normal honey bee behavior and strive to avoid abnormal behavior, as this may be an indication of distress.

The reduction or elimination of pain is also fundamental to performing humane euthanasia. What constitutes a death free of pain requires that how, and even if, the animal experiences pain is understood.[3] Much of our understanding of pain perception comes from mammalian models. Invertebrates do have nociception, or the ability to respond to noxious stimuli.[3,15,16] This ability has been shown in honey bees by measuring the sting extension response following the application of a voltage stimulus.[17] Although the capacity for nociception is a requirement for the ability to experience pain, it is a reflex response and on its own is insufficient evidence.[18] However, in addition to nociception, honey bees demonstrate complex behaviors,[3] and veterinarians should work under the assumption that pain and distress can be experienced by this species until there is scientific evidence that proves otherwise.

The AVMA used a well-defined set of criteria when evaluating the various methods of euthanasia commonly used or recommended in several species under veterinary purview (**Box 1**). These criteria should be considered in the context of the current, and commonly used, methods of euthanasia in North American apiculture as outlined above. The fact that there is not yet sufficient evidence to develop species-specific

---

Box 1
The 14 criteria used for the evaluation of euthanasia methods as quoted from the American Veterinary Medical Association Guidelines for the Euthanasia of Animals: 2020 Edition

"(1) [A]bility to induce loss of consciousness and death with a minimum of pain and distress; (2) time required to induce loss of consciousness; (3) reliability; (4) safety of personnel; (5) irreversibility; (6) compatibility with intended animal use and purpose; (7) documented emotional effect on observers or operators; (8) compatibility with subsequent evaluation, examination, or use of tissue; (9) drug availability and human abuse potential; (10) compatibility with species, age, and health status; (11) ability to maintain equipment in proper working order; (12) safety for predators or scavengers should the animal's remains be consumed; (13) legal requirements; and (14) environmental impacts of the method or disposition of the animal's remains."

From AVMA Guidelines for the Euthanasia of Animals: 2020 Edition. American Veterinary Medical Association.

criteria for honey bee euthanasia does not mean that veterinarians should not work toward meeting these generalized criteria.

The commonly used euthanasia methods presumably use a chemical to bring about death, such as diesel fuel, soapy water, or alcohol. Chemical methods, and in particular, alcohol and formalin, used in invertebrates are reported to work via destruction of the brain and/or major ganglia.[3] Chemical as well as physical methods, such as boiling, freezing, or pithing, are not considered to be humane when used alone.[3] It should be noted that this is the consensus stated in the AVMA guidelines under the methods of euthanasia in captive invertebrates. There are no honey bee-specific guidelines currently available for veterinary medicine, nor does there appear to be research into how the specific current methodologies work in this species.

In general, research into methods of euthanasia of all invertebrates is limited, partially because of the fact that they are typically not covered under animal welfare regulations as are vertebrates.[3,15] The preferred method in insects and other terrestrial invertebrates is to use an inhalant anesthetic, such as isoflurane, sevoflurane, or halothane. CO_2 immobilization, in entomologic research, remains a popular immobilization agent, but remains controversial because of the risk of negative effects, such as convulsion and excitation.[19-21] Anesthesia and immobilization can be followed up with a physical or chemical method as an adjunct to ensure that death has occurred.[3,15] Although this approach may result in a more humane death, it may not be practical or safe under field conditions nor from an economic standpoint. Research into humane euthanasia of invertebrates tends to look at the individual animal.[3,15,22] A colony can contain tens of thousands of honey bees and handling them individually would not only be time-prohibitive but also likely result in undue distress; therefore, euthanasia of honey bees needs to be evaluated at the colony level. Colony euthanasia is further complicated by the fact that the colony contains individuals at various stages of development, which may require different methodologies as well as evaluation to verify death. A future possibility may be to consider a contained system similar to a CO_2 foam distribution system that is used for depopulation of active chicken houses.[23]

Following euthanasia and before disposal, it is important to confirm that death has occurred.[3] Adult honey bees can be checked to ensure they are immobilized and unresponsive to stimuli. More research needs to be done to determine species-specific criteria for verifying death of a colony. These criteria will ideally include a combination of factors as well as factors for evaluating developmental stages in addition to adults.

Psychological impact on the operator, beekeeper, and any observers should not be overlooked. The human-animal bond exists between beekeepers and their colonies and needs to be respected. Communication is essential and should include a discussion of the timing and method of euthanasia and what the beekeepers are likely to observe should they choose to be present. Beekeepers should be notified when death is confirmed, and it may be necessary to offer referral for grief support.[3] Situations in which colonies are mandated to be destroyed because of infectious or foreign pests and diseases may be especially challenging for the beekeeper to accept.

It is imperative that euthanized colonies and associated equipment are disposed of properly to prevent harm to scavenging animals, the environment, and transmission of infectious disease.[3] Prompt disposal is important with respect to honey bees, as colonies in the area will invade and rob a dead colony, putting them at risk for disease transmission and exposure to chemical residues. Depending on the reason for euthanasia and the method chosen, the equipment, and particularly the frames, may not be suitable for reuse. Many states and provinces have specific requirements regarding proper disposal. In the case where destruction must occur by fire, care should be taken to ensure all necessary safety precautions are taken, and the resulting ash should be buried.

SUMMARY

Veterinarians working with honey bees must familiarize themselves with local, state/ provincial, and federal rules and regulations regarding honey bee disease management and control. The appropriate authorities need to be alerted of any case that may potentially fall under these regulations.

There is a current lack of guidelines and standards specific to the humane euthanasia of honey bees. Common methods currently in use likely do not fulfill all requirements for humane euthanasia. There is a need for research into humane methods, as well as a furthering of our understanding of pain perception, signs of distress, unconsciousness and anesthesia, and criteria of confirming death in all life stages within honey bee colonies. However, aspects of euthanasia beyond the methodology can and should still be followed to the highest professional standard as would be done for any animal species.

CLINICS CARE POINTS

- Veterinarians should consult with provincial/state apiarists, extensionists, and technical transfer teams to develop a plan for euthanasia of colonies.

- The method selected should be one that can be performed quickly and with minimal handling of the colony. The veterinarian and beekeeper need to be comfortable with the method chosen.

- Veterinarians should stay up-to-date on research and recommendations regarding the euthanasia of honey bees. As information becomes available, veterinarians can adapt current methodologies to better align them with the guidelines for humane euthanasia.

DISCLOSURE

The authors have nothing to disclose.

REFERENCES

1. Euthanasia – position statement. Canadian Veterinary Medical Association. 2014. Available# at: https://www.canadianveterinarians.net/documents/euthanasia#: ~ : text=The%20Canadian%20Veterinary%20Medical%20Association%20(CVMA)% 20holds%20that%20when%20animals,%2C%20temperament%2C%20and%20 health%20status. Accessed January 1, 2021.
2. Turner PV, Doonan G. Developing on-farm euthanasia plans. Can Vet J 2010; 51(9):1031–4.
3. AVMA guidelines for the euthanasia of animals: 2020 edition. American Veterinary Medical Association; 2020. Available at: https://www.avma.org/sites/default/files/ 2020-01/2020-Euthanasia-Final-1-17-20.pdf. Accessed January 1, 2021.
4. Destruction Protocol for Honey Bee Colonies Found with American Foulbrood (AFB). Ministry of agriculture, food and rural affairs. Available at: http://www. omafra.gov.on.ca/english/food/inspection/bees/destructionprotocol.htm. Accessed May 15, 2021.
5. Module 30: the role of veterinarians in honey bee health. USDA National Veterinary Accreditation Program. Available at: https://nvap.aphis.usda.gov/BEE/ bee0001.php. Accessed May 16, 2021.

6. Killing AFB colonies. The Management Agency National American foulbrood pest management plan. Available at: https://afb.org.nz/killing-colonies/. Accessed May 15, 2021.

7. Managing pests and diseases. BeeAware. Available at: https://beeaware.org.au/code-of-practice/managing-pests-and-diseases. Accessed May 15, 2021.

8. Vidal-Naquet N. Honeybee veterinary medicine: Apis mellifera L. Sheffield, UK: 5m; 2015.

9. Diagnosing and treating American foulbrood in honey bee colonies. Michigan State University, College of Natural Science, Michigan Pollinator Initiative. Available at: https://pollinators.msu.edu/resources/beekeepers/diagnosing-and-treating-american-foulbrood-in-honey-bee-colonies. Accessed May 15, 2021.

10. Honey Bee Diseases: American Foulbrood. Penn State Extension. Available at: https://extension.psu.edu/honey-bee-diseases-american-foulbrood. Accessed May 15, 2021.

11. Beesource. Available at: www.beesource.com/threads. Accessed March 15, 2021.

12. Material safety data sheet. U.S. Department of Labor. Available at: https://www.planetnatural.com/wp-content/uploads/sulfur-fungicide-msds.pdf. Accessed May 15, 2021.

13. How to get rid of a bee hive. WikiHow. Available at: https://www.wikihow.com/Get-Rid-of-a-Beehive. Accessed May 15, 2021.

14. How to kill bees with soapy water. Honey Bee Suite. Available at: www.honeybeesuite.com/how-to-kill-bees-with-soapy-water. Accessed May 15, 2021.

15. Cooper JE. Anesthesia, analgesia, and euthanasia of invertebrates. ILAR J 2011; 52(2):196–204.

16. Murray MJ. Euthanasia. In: Lewbart G, editor. Invertebrate medicine. *2nd Edition*. Iowa: Wiley-Blackwell; 2012.

17. Tedjakumala SR, Aimable M, Giufra M. Pharmacological modulation of aversive responsiveness in honey bees. Front Behav Neurosci 2013;7:221.

18. Elwood RW. Pain and suffering in invertebrates? ILAR J 2011;52(2):175–84.

19. Lewbart GA, Mosley C. Clinical anesthesia and analgesia in invertebrates. J Exot Pet Med 2012;21:59–70.

20. Shen J, Yang P, Zhu X, et al. CO2 anesthesia on Drosophila survival in aging research. Arch Insect Biochem Physiol 2020;103:e21639.

21. Blickenstaff CC. Grasshoppers: effect of CO2 anesthesia. J Econ Entomol 1973; 66(2):538–9.

22. Bennie NAC, Loaring CD, Bennie MMG, et al. An effective method for terrestrial arthropod euthanasia. J Exp Biol 2012;215:4237–41.

23. Gurung S, Hoffman J, Stringfellow K, et al. Depopulation of caged layer hens with a compressed air foam system. Animals 2018;8(1):11.

Moving?

Make sure your subscription moves with you!

To notify us of your new address, find your **Clinics Account Number** (located on your mailing label above your name), and contact customer service at:

Email: journalscustomerservice-usa@elsevier.com

800-654-2452 (subscribers in the U.S. & Canada)
314-447-8871 (subscribers outside of the U.S. & Canada)

Fax number: 314-447-8029

Elsevier Health Sciences Division
Subscription Customer Service
3251 Riverport Lane
Maryland Heights, MO 63043

*To ensure uninterrupted delivery of your subscription, please notify us at least 4 weeks in advance of move.